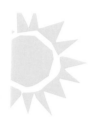

*This book is
presented to*

_____

by

Celebration of **HOPE** Foundation

on behalf of

_____

*111-1445 West Georgia Street Vancouver, B.C. V6G 2T3
Tel: (604) 682-1234 Fax: (604) 682-6004*

HEALERS AT WORK

HEALERS AT WORK

Firsthand Accounts of the Difference
Alternative Healing Makes

PETER DOWNIE

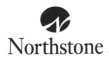

Northstone

Editor: Michael Schwartzentruber
Cover design: Lois Huey-Heck
Consulting art director: Robert MacDonald

Photo credits:
Back cover, Tim McKenna; Wayne Irwin and Flora Litt, Welcome Aboard Photography;
Barbara Bishop, The Photo Company; Rochelle Graham, Lionel Trudel; Jim and Donna
Sinclair, Singleton Photography; Jennifer Jonas, Pierre Gautreau; Kathryn McMorrow,
Jim Harrison; Kelly Walker, V. Tony Hauser; Lois Wilson, Peter Williams.

Northstone Publishing Inc. is an employee-owned company, committed to caring for
the environment and all creation. Northstone recycles, reuses and composts, and en-
courages readers to do the same. Resources are printed on recycled paper and more
environmentally friendly groundwood papers (newsprint), whenever possible. The trees
used are replaced through donations to the Scoutrees For Canada Program. Ten per-
cent of all profit is donated to charitable organizations.

Canadian Cataloguing in Publication Data

Downie, Peter.
      Healers at Work

ISBN 1-55145-080-1
1. Alternative medicine. I. Title
R733.D68 1996   615.5   C96-910434-0

Published by Northstone Publishing Inc.

Northstone

Printed in Canada by Best Book Manufacturers

Dedication

This is for Jan who shall be forever an inspiration in my life.

એ

Acknowledgments

I feel blessed to have had a friend like Gary Katz for over 20 years. His humor, wise advice and gentleness are an invisible but integral part of these pages.

Marlene McArdle is a valued friend and colleague. This couldn't have been done without her experience, dedication, and skill.

And finally, I feel lucky to know France, Myles, and Sean who continue to show me the possibilities of life.

Table of Contents

Preface

A part of me, I must confess, was nervous about tackling the subject of healing – mainly because it is a landscape increasingly littered with slick not to mention impressive but impossible promises of miracle cures specifically aimed at people whose fear of illness and death makes them all the more gullible and desperate.

Given the excesses of the frenzied marketplace of "health" and "better living" products, I want you to understand that there are no promises or gimmicks or get-well-quick schemes contained in these pages.

I also believe you deserve to know my definition of healing before we begin and I've wondered how best to express the critical distinction between curing and healing. To that end, it seems to me that while a medical condition can sometimes be cured, the human condition – individually and collectively – is almost always in need of some healing.

This kind of healing is about reaching an emotional, physical, and/or spiritual equanimity with the demands and complexities of modern life in North America. It's a healing which takes for granted the elaborate interconnectedness and value of the heart and soul and mind and body all striving together to reach that elusive moment of a true and profound sense of well-being. It's a healing which battles against what writer and philosopher Sir Laurens Van der Post calls the modern crisis of feeling "unknown in the universe." This is a healing which connects us not only to those we love, but also to life, with all the joy and sadness and mystery it contains.

The people you are about to meet have been chosen carefully. They are the real thing, working at helping others to genuinely heal. And while neither I nor they would claim that any one of them has the perfectly packaged and complete answer, I'm convinced each contributes a very important piece of the healing puzzle. Their survival in our "get-whatever-you-want-now, drive-thru, disposable" society is a clear measure of the growing interest many of us have in taking back some control over our own health and well-being.

One of the intriguing aspects for me as this work progressed was how different, on the surface, each of them was from the others. But then, as we started to probe more deeply the healing process, I came to understand just how much they all have in common. It's ironic that while "process" is the best word to describe how each approaches healing and is the common denominator that clearly draws all these healers together, it is precisely that "process" which makes every healing journey unique and personal. We all must find our own way of reaching answers that make sense.

As much as we might like it to be so, healing can't be bought for any amount of money. There are no shortcuts or tricks or deals to be made. It doesn't wear a white coat and we can't make a yearly appointment to heal. If we reach a point in our lives when it becomes important to heal, we must accept that the "process" simply isn't possible without our careful and constant involvement.

There are other words you'll notice that are common to these healers: respect, energy, integrity, safety, community, loving, caring, sharing, intention, hope, justice, and honesty. These are a far cry from "extra billing, user fees, federal/provincial jurisdiction, transfer payments, opting in, opting out" – the usual language dominating Canada's continuing health care debate.

But then, healing has little to do with the billions we spend on drugs every year and it's a long way from just the practice of medicine. Granted, that practice has been revolutionized by technology, much of it helpful and worthwhile. But our high-tech wizardry has also created situations in which our "know-how" has raced ahead of our ability to make reasoned judgments about the ethics and morality of its application.

We pay a very steep price for getting ahead of our hearts and I think I've learned that the heart is where any healing process truly begins. You're about to read of people who can find healing in death, who choose not to run but to learn from the darkness of life, who heal others by offering safety and compassion, who heal the heart's pain at life's end by celebrating memory, and who discover purpose and meaning and belonging by listening to the richness of silence.

Looking back now, my almost immediate "yes" to this project seems strange, if not foolhardy given the fact that I had spent the past 25 years in front of either a radio microphone or a television camera. The explanation? I think I just knew this would be time well spent. It turned out I was right and my modest hope now, as you begin to turn these pages and to meet these healers, is that you too will find something worthwhile here.

I want to thank each of these healers for spending time with me and for patiently telling me what they do and how they do it so well. My appreciation goes as well to Mike Schwartzentruber whose skill as an editor kept me upright and balanced during my first shaky steps in a new world.

Chapter 1
THE DANCE OF LIFE

The Healing Journey   *Kelly Walker*

❧

❧

The ancient Greek poet Aeschylus wrote, "In our sleep, pain which we cannot forget falls drop by drop upon the heart until against our will, in our own despair, comes wisdom through the awful grace of God." Kelly Walker is one of those people in whom there has been much pain. You recognize that about him almost immediately. But in addition to the reward of wisdom Aeschylus promised, Kelly Walker is proof that healing and a sense of rightful balance in one's life can also be achieved by making it through those dark periods.

Actually, "making it through" sounds too much like simply surviving the inevitable moments of darkness or depression which each of us is faced with in life. Kelly Walker thinks we shouldn't run from the darkness, that for our health we must embrace those episodes, explore them, touch them, feel them, smell them, taste them, and, in the end, become as familiar and comfortable with them as we are with our moments of joy.

He is a Dominican priest who left his Order and a husband who left his marriage, but he is very much a man who has achieved, through all that pain, an understanding of what it means to be a human being embarked on a journey of healing. After spending a little time with him, I sense that he is a powerful healer.

I've been thinking of how a professional photographer or visual artist learns early on the value of playing with shadows, understanding the richness that's revealed when dark dances with light. It is a much harder but equally valuable lesson in life, one that many of us, I'm afraid, never quite grasp.

❧

PD: Tell me about the journey that took you from a place where you felt some comfort in the church, to a place where you felt so very uncomfortable in it.

KW: Well, the church saga became uncomfortable for a lot of reasons. I think, at the root of it, we were deceived. I was part of the revolution in terms of the Second Vatican Council. It became clear as the 1970s progressed that this Pope was opting for a 1950s-style of religious expression and that a revitalized and evolving faith-style suitable for the year 2,000 wasn't an option. We'd been preparing our congregations and our people around the world for the year 2,000 and it wasn't going to happen.

And so we felt deceived. I was going to say disillusioned. I think that's okay, to lose your illusions, but we were deceived. The institution was starting to re-center on itself and the revolution just wasn't going to happen. As a result, I began to go through a deep, inner depression around the issue of people's needs, needs that we were able to meet but that we weren't allowed to meet. We were considered, not just bad, but evil, I think.

We had created, in our little Dominican community here, one of the first mixed communities in the Order. We had women living with us and women preaching and women involved in ministry, and I was told to disallow that. I was also told by the Order in Rome, not because of the Order but because of its relationship

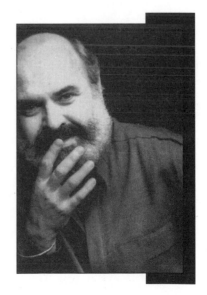

with the Roman authority, that we had better get back into line and go back to our traditional forms.

Well, it would have been like putting toothpaste back into the tube. It was cruel, and frankly, stupid, and they're reaping the consequences of that now. Somebody said to me a while ago that he had left the church and I said, "No, I think the church has left you."

PD: Well, I wanted to ask you who you think betrayed whom, when you look back at it now. Do you feel betrayed?

KW: Yes, absolutely. And a whole generation of us does. If it was just me I could get over it and say it's just...

PD: Something in you.

KW: That it was just something in me. But I know for a fact that it's a whole generation of us – those of us who are in our 50s and 60s. I'm 54 now and I think that the future of the church has been embraced by neoconservatives and frightened homophobic males. They are frightened of their boys' club being invaded.

I was at Notre Dame in the 1960s when it became co-ed and the boys at Notre Dame went through the same thing. They got over it, though, probably because there had been some titillation. The Roman people have their titillation in their boys' club, so they don't want it invaded by women who would bring wonderful balance and question and harmony.

PD: You have a real sense of that dilemma now, but, when it was going on, did you have a hard time identifying all of this, what was wrong?

KW: No, I understood it.

PD: You did?

KW: I understood it. As the organization became more misogynous, it became more and more difficult to be there. Part of my internal breakdown, I think, came also from a terrible discrepancy. It was a huge issue of integrity. Sexual truths were never allowed to happen or to be told. But sexual reality is not a big, bad bogeyman; it's just a normal part of being a human being. So people were living deceitful lives and there was this huge, huge fear that the tables would be turned by the women having power; women are more inclined to seek out and tell the truth than males.

PD: Most of the traditional, medical establishment types I've spoken with dismiss the Christian idea of there being nobility in suffering as silly. I don't know if what you went through then you would characterize as noble, but you do incorporate it into the healer that you've become. You've said even just the telling of the story is a form of healing. How do you understand that now?

KW: It's interesting, because I have friends who have stayed in the Roman church and who continue to suffer and I don't feel at this stage that it's necessary. It wouldn't have been noble for me to stay there.

But I think the suffering I went through there had some nobility to it because it helped me understand and have compassion for people's journeys. Later, I think it helped me in that it provided a frame of reference; it made stupid things really look stupid and sensible things really make sense.

I think one of the things I discovered was that, for myself, I didn't have the right to stay there and use my good energy and my good life to fight for something that was just not going to change. At some point, I think, there's nobility in saying, "Enough of this! This isn't something that's really of benefit to people." And I began to see, with my gifts and my talents, that I was going to be of more benefit to this generation outside the church. I do the same stuff now, I just don't do it under the auspices of a dysfunctional organization.

PD: But there is, you think, suffering that is of benefit?

KW: Absolutely. I think there's suffering that is of benefit to the individual because it's a necessary part of what goes on in the human dance. In the dance of the earth, everything that has an up, has a down. The wave is up, over the line, under the line, and back up. I think that's an important law of physics. It's an important law of what goes on on this earth with everything.

So the suffering, which sometimes is repose or pit or under the line, depression maybe, can be really salvific. Salvation is a theological word for health. I think there is something in the essence of the human dance that is about, not just happiness, but also sadness. It's the light and the dark, it's the shadow and the radiant side.

PD: The balance.

KW: Yes. And I think they both happen whether we program them or not. Our decision in living life is to see whether or not we're going to value those down times. Now, we've been taught not to value them in this generation. We've been taught to medicate them, or we've been taught just to bandage them or eradicate them. Look what we do with death! If we go into the depths and listen to what's going on, and get words and icons for it – whatever goes on down there – then I think it can be of great value to us, even salvific.

I just wrote to the first friend I ever had. We were little kids together in Walkerton and I haven't talked to her since we were 20! But I met her nephew in Saskatchewan last week and so I wrote to her. I said that my life has been wonderful, but that in the eyes of a lot of onlookers, it would be horrible.

I've had losses, I've left institutions – the Roman church and marriage – but I think those losses were part of what I have to do. They are part of an uncovering of who Kelly is, what this embodied soul is about.

I think I've lost my soul several times, or almost lost my soul several times, in doing what others have needed me to do for them to be okay, or in doing what I perceived I needed to do for my mom or my dad or various institutions to be happy. But I think when the breakdowns came, they came because, somehow, I wasn't living in harmony with myself. They came as a very important juncture in my life, to help me realize that if I wanted to reclaim who I was – in my case to claim it for the first time – then I'd have to take some of the stands that would lead me out of those situations.

PD: But understanding the light and the dark of that "human dance," you must arrive at a pretty interesting definition of healing.

KW: I think healing, somehow, has something to do with the process of going through the kaleidoscope of pits, with guidance if you can find it, until you get to some kind of new stability, or new integrity. Integrity. I think that's what it's about.

PD: But it's physical, it's emotional.

KW: It's everything. Nothing is just emotional. Nothing is just mental. Nothing is just physical in us. We're an eco-system.

PD: We forgot that for a long time, didn't we?

KW: I think so. I think we forgot it after Descartes and the Gnostics. There's a whole Gnostic disease that goes on in society. It's very strong in religion right now with the charismatic movement. And American religion is Gnostic. It's very sick. It forgets that we are multifaceted and that no one facet of us functions without the other. Alexander Lowen, the father of bioenergetics, talks about it, for example, in his book *Depression and the Body*.

I'm pretty big physically, but I'm bigger than I look because I've got all kinds of energy around me and I'm interconnected! Part of my reality is my interconnection with everybody that I've ever connected with. In the church, we used to call that the communion of saints, a link with everything that was and everything that will be. So I'm a much bigger entity than I appear. And now that they're discovering all of these new galaxies and things, I think we're part of all that, too.

You know, traditional psychiatry seems to deal with the mind, the subconscious, the unconscious, and I don't think it's enough. I think we're much bigger than that.

PD: What does that mean in terms of your work as a healer?

KW: There's an underlying groundwork that I live with. For anybody who is going through a dark time, or what I call a *tardemah* – which is usually why people come to a healer – there is a mystical or dream dimension involved. So everything is involved: their dream, their imagination, their sexuality, their food intake and digestion, their left-brain right-brain mechanical functioning, their productivity in society, their faith, their spirituality, their oxygen intake, their breathing – all of that, their whole ecosystem.

All the parts of the ecosystem go into a dark time when we're in a dark time. And somehow, in order to pull us beyond the dark time or *tardemah*, it's necessary to re-stimulate everything. And generally, when you're in a point of darkness or confusion, you can't do that all by yourself. So that's when you have to go to the shaman, or the holy person, or the healer to get some kind of energy for that next step. It's one of the reasons why it's very important for the healer to have excellent energy and to be connected to all of the sources of things.

PD: When we were kids, the idea that a depression might have something to do with what you eat for breakfast, that there is an important nutritional factor in depression, would have simply been dismissed.

KW: Absolutely. The depression was dismissed, first of all! When you and I were kids, you weren't supposed to have it. "Cheer up! Pull your socks up and get on with it!" we were told. And if you were depressed, it was never valued until you hit mid-life or until you were an adult. If you were a kid and you were depressed, you were just a bum or lazy or something was wrong with you.

By the time you got to mid-life, then you called it a nervous depression and you were sent away to an institution of some kind where they gave you shock treatment or they medicated you and made you a zombie. We have never valued a depression or a breakdown. What we said was, "Whatever you do, get over it." And for the most part, those who were so heavily medicated never really came back. They were not allowed to do so by their family or their workplace or whatever.

PD: Could that mean that we also didn't value or understand healing?

KW: We didn't understand healing. I think we valued...

PD: Cure.

KW: Absolutely. We valued cure or what we considered to be cure. What we valued was numbing or eradication and in Western medicine we've done that; we've cauterized. If something is wrong, we just cut it out.

Oriental medicine, on the other hand, would say that if there's distress in the system, what we have to do is re-balance the system, rebalance the energies. That happens through acupuncture, shiatsu or moxabustion, or some other therapy that will restore that balance. The shamans did it through exorcisms, some way of rebalancing the energy. All we did was cut it out with a knife or with a drug.

PD: Is there a healer within each of us?

KW: Yes. Meister Eckhart, who was a 14th-century Dominican, says that each one of us is a mystic. In the same way, each one of us is a healer.

I believe that everything on this earth can self-heal. But generally, when we're in a state of breakdown, we don't have the energy necessary to do it, so we have to get it from somebody else.

We have to get the inspiration from somebody else. I think I only heal if I have the healing power, which is already within me, stirred up. So I don't think it's you who heals me; I think you remind my ecosystem that it can do it. Or you help my ecosystem get into a situation where it can begin the process of self-healing.

PD: So shiatsu massage, for example, will inspire one's own inner knowledge, if I can put it that way?

KW: Yes, definitely.

PD: Do you know how that works?

KW: I think it "re-minds" us.

I've never been as conscious of that as I have been in the last few years. I had a hunch that my healing was going to require some kind of body stuff. I can remember lying on the floor at the shiatsu clinic that I went to first, and saying I could be a corpse in the same outfit at a funeral home! And I thought, isn't this wonderful; somebody's going to come in and restimulate my system by touch. I didn't realize, initially, that it was going to make me breathe again, but shiatsu makes you breathe. I realized that, somehow, it was going to help my system remember what health was like and then it would want to stay there.

I think when we go into disease, we embrace a state that isn't really us. We embrace a state that is "other." That's why, traditionally, in native societies, exorcism was done: to get that evil spirit, that "other" out of the person. And once I realize who I am again and realize that it feels good and that there's pleasure in it, that's when I embrace the healing process. My ecosystem reminds, or "re-minds," itself that that's where I should be and it starts to function.

PD: What do you mean by "learning to breathe again?"

KW: When we go into a depression or a state of sadness, we start to breathe shallowly, we almost stop breathing. Breathing can stimulate rebirth. One of the main things that an expectant mother has to do when learning birthing techniques is learn to breathe again.

PD: And, of course, our breathing can signal the approach of death.

KW: That's right, because we're getting ready to go to another state or phase. We can access the energy that's needed to get us beyond a depression by stimulating the breathing again and we can do it in any way we want.

We can do it through bioenergetic therapy; we can do it through shiatsu or yoga which are wonderful; we can do it through aerobics, by just walking and moving our arms. I sometimes get people to put a little "rebounder" in their rooms. I'm thinking of getting one here and just jumping up and down; it stimulates the breathing.

PD: In North America, it seems we've been seduced by

consumerism, the idea that somebody else is going to do it for us.

KW: Absolutely.

PD: But you're saying it's in us.

KW: In North America, if you come to me and pay me for healing, I need you to stay! It's absurd, but I think that's what happens in a lot of cases – especially when I, as therapist or whatever, can charge it to a public health plan. I can just keep it going as long as I want. I have had people come to me who have been seeing a psychiatrist for years and I wonder, "Why were you in therapy?" Perhaps it was to help the psychiatrist's ego.

I think the main function of the healer, on the other hand, is to try to help the person go away. "Please go away! You've been here long enough!"

I always thought you went into a psychotherapeutic process to get out of it!

PD: But if healing is also a "process," does it have an end? Can you reach the point of being healed?

KW: I think so. But then you wait for the next thing to come along. I think we have a number of breakdowns, anything that's alive does. At that point, you might go to another healer.

When I was leaving the Order, I somehow needed a woman, so I went to an older woman who helped me. When I was dealing with other issues, issues of sexuality in my life, I needed a male. When I dealt with issues of inner turmoil, I needed a holy man or somebody who had a sense of

God. I think I need my healer to have some sense of the "other," but not necessarily to be attached to a religious institution. Sometimes I find that the healers who are attached to an institution have a prejudice for the institution.

PD: It occurs to me that one of the things which is easy to say – we all repeat it and it seems particularly apt for your story – is that what we do is not who we are. In your healing work, have you seen people struggle with that distinction?

KW: Somebody in the recovery movement in the United States says that we've become "human doings" and I think that's exactly what's happened in North America. We have valued "doing" and we have devalued "being" so the contemplative values are hugely dismissed.

Ten years ago, I left a period of absolute doing. I was a good priest. No parish is going to hire a priest or a minister who is healthy. They want a crazy workaholic so that they can get their money's worth out of him or her. If you say, "I'm sorry, I reserve time for prayer," well, forget it. "We want you in there working!" So if you're out of the office you're in trouble and if you're in the office you're in trouble because you're not doing whatever it is they expect you to be doing. Many people go crazy with this attitude. Your self-definition is based on doing.

Most of my major work has been with people in ministry, in health care, in education, and in social work. Most of those people are driven crazy by "doing," but they're expected to "do"! They've got to be doing, and if they're not doing, they're not valued, which is worse even than not being paid.

Too often they are valued by virtue of the inner diseases they've got, their co-dependency needs, which most people in those professions have. They need to be valued. And if that value is visible, then they feel as though they're somebody and that they're going to be all right.

PD: But can healing also work with a "human doing"?

KW: Oh yes. Usually with a "human doing," though, it takes a breakdown first, because the "human doing" will keep on doing until he or she cracks. Sometimes it's too late. Too many of us in our generation have died of heart attack or cancer or accidents that haven't been that at all. They've been heart attacks and cancer and accidents sure, but that's not really what was going on. What was going on in many cases, is what I call "soul loss."

They can no longer "do" and have revved themselves up to the point of disappearance. And so at some point their ecosystem just says, "Screw you. Die." I don't know if there's a "next time around," but I think that if there is, that's the stuff they're going to have to deal with – that somehow in the dance of life they didn't embrace their soul, their being.

PD: I'm sure everyone has people who they've lost through cancer or heart attack and it certainly wasn't anything intentional on the part of the soul that was lost.

KW: Absolutely. But I think interiorly that's probably what goes on. Their system just says, "I can't do this anymore."

My own 1981 breakdown was very visible and had suicidal aspects to it as well. My car was driving off the road, I was trying to escape. I started to cry. I cried relentlessly for about a year. I couldn't stop crying, couldn't stop throwing up, couldn't stop the diarrhea, couldn't stop withdrawing.

So my breakdown saved my life in some ways, and helped me to recover who I was.

PD: It got your attention.

KW: Yes. It was a long process because I'd been a "human doing" for so long. To suddenly start valuing my being was absolutely novel! Isn't that crazy? To think that I lived in a monastery and yet I got to be so busy there. You can become busy anywhere. The busiest people I know are farmers, who we tend to idealize as having a wonderful, contemplative life.

PD: There's a romantic notion about life in the country.

KW: Oh yes. So I think we all dig our own grave, however we want to do that.

But the recovery of being is extremely difficult. After a long period of intense doing, sometimes the only way out is to stop. Generally it takes a firing, or being caught, or a breakdown of some kind. I think it takes something of that magnitude to recover some people's being. Now often, they don't pay attention to it and so they die or they go back into the doing. You see, in our society, we've very seldom looked upon "doing" as a possible disease.

PD: It's achievement.

KW: Absolutely. Your parents are happy, you know. The institutions you work for are delighted. But they've got a sick baby on their hands.

PD: But you know what's interesting is that the people who are still "doing," those who continue to generate and provide the fuel for that system to continue, dismiss this as New Age whereas, in fact, it's the oldest age possible! This wisdom is from...

KW: Eternity.

PD: Our ancient past.

KW: Yes. Anne Wilson Schaef has a good book called *The Addictive Organization*. It describes what happens when the head of an organization is an addict, whether it's of alcohol, drugs, work, or perfectionism. When that happens, the head of an organization becomes a crazy maker and everybody in the organization is forced to live as though the emperor had clothes. Everybody in the organization takes on the emperor's disease.

The child of an alcoholic usually ends up being crazier than the alcoholic. Often, when we're in a system that's crazy, we don't even recognize that it's crazy because it has become so normal. We function the way it wants us to function.

PD: But does healing require then that you can't remain in that organization? Or can you survive it from some base of health?

KW: Sometimes you've got to leave it. I think it depends on how sick it is. Or if you decide you have the strength – which, if you're sick, you don't usually have – you can stay and try to transform it from within. And some institutions are valuable enough that it's worthwhile doing that.

PD: You see, I'm afraid some people might dismiss this idea of healing as a luxury. It's very nice to think of it that way, but I have obligations.

KW: I remember saying to my stepfather, "You can have a priest in a casket or you can have a son who's healthy." He immediately phoned the funeral home!

PD: I don't believe that!

KW: Your faith isn't very deep, my son! But that's what happens. You can be dead because you can die! Or you can come to health and make some changes.

If you have a job, you can probably get a job. You might not be able to live in the palace you lived in previously, but maybe that was what was killing you.

Now this painting here is of a vision I had on the day I made my final vows. It wasn't a dream. It was a vision of a big grand piano in a big room with windows, on the east coast somewhere, with water crashing up against the rocks.

I got quite frightened and went to one of the Brothers in the monastery and said, "I really think I should leave. I think this is a vision that's telling me I shouldn't be here." And he assured me it was just a temptation. I know now it wasn't and I should have paid attention to it. But we don't pay attention to our visions or our dreams because we have been taught that they're not real. Actually, they are real, but in this environment they're not considered to be real.

One of the things my psychiatrist got me to do when I left the Order was to buy that grand piano. The nuns lent me some money – I paid them back – and I bought it.

Well, you can't have a grand piano in a basement apartment so I had to get a snazzy place for $1,350 a month!

The piano had a great apartment, but I had to work at the bar at night, do therapy during the day, and give concerts whenever I could. One day I came home and I looked at the piano and I said, "You lucky thing! You're sitting here all day in this lovely place and I'm working myself to death to pay rent so you can have a lovely home and I'm never here to enjoy you!"

Well, that's what people do. So often, in their work, they put all of the value on what they get from the money they're paid. My confrère Matthew Fox, in a book called *The Reinvention of Work*, talks about our work which is our "great work." "What am I in this universe for?" Everyone of us is here for something and we've got to have our antennae out to figure out what that is. Sometimes our "job" has to do with our "work," but sometimes it doesn't.

Sometimes, what the breakdown allows us to do is to rediscover or to discover for the first time what our "work" is. I think the breakdown generally comes from the "job." I've never seen a breakdown come because of the "work." And so, very often, because all of the stuff around the job is related to the breakdown, I have to leave the job and go on this journey. But we're scared to do that.

PD: I was just going to say it takes a lot of courage to heal this way, doesn't it?

KW: Yes.

PD: So is part of your healing to give people that courage?

KW: I believe so. Some of it's been through modeling. I think one of the important roles of the elder or the healer is to tell his or her story, to provide people with some mythology they can hang their hat on while they're going through their own journey. I usually tell people ancient stories to help them, and I tell them mine – although it too is getting more and more ancient.

PD: And it's also the way we know those ancient stories. Maybe we have always known, instinctively, the healing power of storytelling and that's why people through the ages have taken the time to pass them along.

KW: That's the reality of Jesus of Nazareth. I think he has mythological value in that he becomes another fundamental myth that we need. The Greeks had all kinds of myths to hang onto. Jung and Freud just explored those myths. That's all they did. They explored the stories.

Jesus of Nazareth provides another story as valid and as important for humanity. His time in the desert was a time of clarification, of going crazy. The Devil was putting before him pseudo-selves – that he should embrace them – and he said "no." But he went crazy with that. Kazantzakis portrays that very well in *The Last Temptation of Christ.* Well, we all go crazy. When we go through those major times, we're supposed to go crazy and it's helpful to me to look at Jesus going crazy!

After his baptism in the Jordan, which was a big deal, he would have been in the bad books of his rabbinical friends and of his family. He left traditional orthodox Judaism and followed John the Baptist and embraced a radical reform away from the synagogue and the Temple.

And it says that after the baptism into the religion of John, Jesus was led by the spirit into the desert where he was tempted for 40 days and 40 nights. The Israelites, after they escaped from Egypt, went into the desert for 40 years and that's where their self-definition came from, in that struggle to figure out who they were. And Jesus of Nazareth then goes into the desert for 40 days and 40 nights and goes crazy.

The Bible says – and this is an important aspect of the healing – that God sent angels to comfort him. Well, I think that's precisely what goes on. I think that in the process of our 40 days and 40 nights – our Lent – the Creator sends angels. Our angels are here, they're around us. Those healing energies that are part of us are there, but we have to trust them.

Most of us don't embrace deserts. We certainly don't go looking for them. We are usually sent, by the spirit, into a desert. But in that desert is all the stuff that we need, I think, to grow through that *tardemah*, that dark time. Then we emerge at the other end, generally new, changed. Something's different. We let go of some things.

PD: Is there an essential attribute, such as openness, that a healer must possess?

KW: I think there are probably a couple. One is integrity. I think God, or creation, or whatever that power is, heals despite the insanity of the healer. But I think it's helpful if there's integrity in the healer, because he or she has to be somehow in touch with all of the healing forces of the universe. It's important that that person be open to those forces, but I don't think he or she has to be perfect in any way. "Open" is probably the best word for what the healer needs to be, because healing comes through, not by, him or her. I think the universe or the Creator is the healer. I think it's

God's dream that we be in health and some of us have the gift of channeling that. It is a gift.

Half the psychiatrists in this town don't have it. They wanted to become a psychiatrist to make money or to work out their own stuff. There are lots of them I wouldn't send anybody to. A healer could be a zany old woman in the center of downtown who's got the gift of healing and the only thing she does might be to talk to somebody on the phone. Healing doesn't just happen in an office and it doesn't just come with a bill attached to it. It's got nothing to do with that. So some people who are professionals might have the gift of healing, but a whole lot of them don't.

PD: But there's a responsibility that goes along with that gift. Once you recognize you have the gift, it must be a burden as well as a joy.

KW: Absolutely, yes.

PD: So what do you do with it?

KW: In my case, I've had to learn how to channel it. At this stage of my life, I don't want to do it one-on-one very often. I think the place I have to do it right now is on the concert stage, singing and talking. And I never, until I wrote my first book, *Loss of Soul*, had a sense that it would have anything to do with writing. I never thought I could write. Maybe I can't! But people buy it and want it, so that's a sign to me that something's being released through that.

PD: There's such a hunger for healing, isn't there?

KW: Amazing hunger. One of the things people say after the concerts is, "We were healed. I came out of there a different person than when I went in. Something healing has gone on."

One of the things that music does, I think, is send vibrations through our whole ecosystem. When I sit down at a piano and play and sing, something much bigger than me happens. I don't understand that, but that's what I hear.

PD: I've been reading Lance Morrow's eloquent memoir *Heart*. He's already had heart attacks and bypass operations and he is only in his 50s. He writes about the cause of heart problems and quotes experts as telling him that it's not smoking, it's not diet, it's what they call "joyless striving" that's causing many of the problems. So in the mix of healing, does there have to be a willingness to be joyful?

KW: One of my dearest friends said to me the other day, "I don't know why I live because I don't really have joy in anything. I just feel resigned to live."

PD: Condemned to life, almost.

KW: I said, "I feel so sad to hear you say that. I want to help you." I don't know how I'm going to help him, but I don't want him to stay there. I can't make him do this, but I want him to delight in his work. And if he doesn't delight in his work, then he should leave it. But we feel condemned to those things.

Often, we feel condemned to relationships. We're getting better and we've learned that it's okay sometimes to leave a relationship, but generally, if we don't go through the healing, we reembrace the same relationship. We marry the same person over and over again.

PD: It's funny how we've come to see joy as being selfish.

KW: I have difficulty talking about pleasure because it frightens people. I was in Saskatoon last week and I was getting people to do some stuff with their bodies – to stretch and breathe – and I had this very angry, Germanic Saskatchewan teacher come up to me and say, "I think you should know that we don't do childish things out here." He said, "As you saw, some of us left while you were doing that."

I just thanked him for telling me that. I figured I'm not going to fight this one, it's generations of toxicity. He was threatened by pleasure. Don't do anything that will allow the child in me to emerge. We don't allow silly. We don't allow pleasure. We don't allow fun. We're very Presbyterian, no matter who we are.

We are a very joyless society and we look for pseudo-pleasure, but then, we've got pseudomodels. We've got Michael Jackson and Madonna. I see icons of Marilyn Monroe and I just want to die! Why would we make an icon of her? We have icons of pseudohumans, of people who didn't embrace their life.

PD: Which is critical to healing?

KW: Absolutely. How can you heal if you're not allowing pleasure energy or joyful energy to come through your laughter? Generally, when we go into dark times, we avoid all those things. We tend to embrace pseudopleasures, such as drinking or eating to excess.

PD: How important is God to you as a healer?

KW: That's an interesting question because I'm having a hard time with her! I'm not having any trouble with God as God. I'm having a great deal of trouble with God as embraced by the religions.

PD: So it's true that God hates religion?

KW: Oh yea. Meister Eckhart used to say, "God deliver me from God."

I have no trouble with God being the energy source and ground of all of our beings. Every time a new galaxy is discovered, or something like that, I realize I don't even understand the end of the block! I guess I think of God more and more as Creator. I probably put a face on it just because that's what we do. I don't dismiss any of the mythology that the Judeo-Christian heritage gives me. I treasure it.

I treasure the Catholic tradition which is enormous and open despite the political forces that want to close it. Protestantism is very small and closed compared to it, except as it is expressed by people such as Paul Tillich and some of the radical Protestant left.

I think that God is at the base of all this, but I just don't feel I need to define his or her face, or whatever, at this time. I just trust.

Meister Eckhart would say that we dwell within God. I was raised to think that God dwells within me, which makes me the center of the universe. But I dwell within the mystery of God, so I live my life trusting that God is there and part of it.

I think I'm probably more of a believer now than I ever

was when I would have defined myself as a this or a that. I'm still on their books as an Anglican priest. As one of my cousins says, I'm on their books but off their radar. And because I've told the truth about my sexuality and because I am in a relationship with a man right now, and have been for some time, I can't function as a priest in that church. I can, if I hide it all, but I'm not willing to hide it. So I can't be a *bona fide* healer under their auspices.

I'm not sure I want to be part of any institution that doesn't embrace truth. I'm still figuring that one out because I love the church. I have a great love for the church, but I'm not sure the church embraces God. I think God is willing to embrace the church. Calvin talks about *l'eglise visible* and *l'eglise invisible*, the visible church and the invisible church. I'm just not sure right now if the church, as we find it today, is the church.

Chapter 2
ODE TO JOY

The Healing Music of *Jennifer Jonas*

❧

I'm told that some of the people around us will probably die within hours.

Even on a palliative care floor of a downtown Toronto hospital, this is an uncomfortable piece of information. While a visitor such as myself can hardly imagine how difficult it must be for the medical professionals to surrender, to raise, in effect, the white flag in the battle against age and/or disease, I'm sitting with someone whose work is just beginning. Someone trained to ease the obvious pain and sorrow of the patient and the family by suggesting something quite remarkable. No drugs, no high-tech wizardry and no medical tour de force. *She simply offers music.*

Her name is Jennifer Jonas and I watch her enter a situation of high drama and great emotion as family members gather awkwardly around the deathbed of their mother. As a music therapist, Ms. Jonas is armed only with her guitar, her warmth, and her gentle nature. Within moments of starting to sing Amazing Grace, *she has brought this family together in a way that is clearly comforting and reassuring in a time of such acute pain.*

Part of the healing she performs on this floor is helping people face the end, by coaxing their lives to come full circle. With the skill of Ms. Jonas, music not only opens the doors to the past, celebrating the life that has been, but it also stands up to the sorrow of the present and anxiety about the future.

Beethoven once wrote that music was a higher revelation than philosophy. I think that Jennifer Jonas, and all those she has touched, would agree.

❧

JJ: The average stay here, Peter, is six weeks. What's very important for me, in my therapeutic practice, is to develop a relationship, to develop a trust, so that when I sing to people they can trust me to release some of their emotions or some of the memories that have been very meaningful to them. I want to do that to increase their self-identity, their sense of who they've been in their life, their sense that they've been loved. So I encourage their trust so that they're free to talk with me. If they don't want to talk, that's their option; I can just sing.

PD: I noticed with Margaret that you remembered a song that her mother would sing to her. Was she reluctant at first to bring back those kinds of memories?

JJ: Yes. With a lot of patients, you come in, you don't know this person, and they're not going to give you all their memories. So you start by singing their favorite songs. From that, and my presence – I'm warm and kind to them and unconditionally accepting of them...

PD: And you're not poking and prodding them.

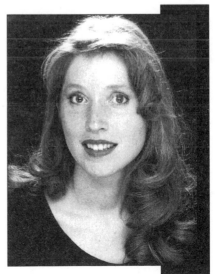

JJ: Right. I'm not related to their pain or their illness. I'm related to positive feelings, memories that bring them a sense of peace and happiness. Sometimes I work with families who tell me they're upset at the doctors – I think, because their loved one is dying and the doctors cannot offer a cure. So I come in and I offer music. They are so pleased that through the music I can offer a sense of peace or happiness to their loved one.

PD: You see happiness?

JJ: Yes. When Margaret was singing along with me, I think she felt good.

PD: And her friends had great smiles, too, when they were singing along. It's almost like a community.

JJ: Yes.

PD: Like an instant community.

JJ: Created by the music.

Often, I will encourage people in the room to get involved with the singing. Barbara is another patient and her two grandchildren are here so what I'll probably do, when I visit with Barbara today, is get them involved by singing children's songs. In that way, I'm indirectly giving something of the grandchildren to the grandmother.

I think of one instance where I worked with a father who was dying. He had two very young children. I could sense that the family relationships were strained and I never heard words of love spoken outright. So I used music to speak of the love the children had for the father.

One day, I went in and the children were there and I said, "You guys sing along with me, I know you know this song." So we sang, "I love you, you love me, we're a happy family..." The little boys looked at daddy and they sang, "I love you, you love me...," which was so true and something the dad needed to hear. He was going to die within a couple of days. And his wife, I think, needed to hear that too. I remember, she sat on the chair and just watched them with a sense of love, taking in that moment and treasuring it, because she knew their moments together were going to be very few.

PD: Now you couldn't, I don't think, walk into a situation like that without a guitar, as a "regular" therapist, and just say, "It's time you people told each other some things."

JJ: Right.

PD: There's something about the music that is the vehicle for it. Do you know what that is?

JJ: Well, first, the words fit with the song. When I start a song, the words are there, so it's almost like I'm feeding these words into their lips.

I also did this with a couple. This woman was dying very young, at 39. Her husband had a hard time, I could sense, expressing his love. But he asked me one night to sing *The Rose* to his wife. So I thought, "Jen, he wants to tell her of his love."

"Some say love, it is a river..."

So I sang that song as a gift from him to her, and the words were not mine, but his, to his wife.

And you're right, I couldn't use my own words. I think that would be more offensive, because who am I to say that. But the song can.

Music is related to beauty and harmony and these songs

are beautiful. What you've created is an atmosphere of love and warmth, friendship and caring through the music, and then through the words.

PD: I don't suppose anybody really understands why music has that impact.

JJ: I've been researching that recently. As a music therapist, I'm constantly seeing the therapeutic effects of music. I work with autistic children, I work with developmentally delayed adults, and here with terminally ill patients, and I'm constantly seeing the transformations that people undergo with the music. Ted Andrews, who wrote *Sacred Sounds*, says everyone is musical. Everyone holds the gift of music within them. So I can work with almost everyone. I have found that music touches our souls, our inner self. It touches deeply, more deeply than words, more deeply than concepts.

I have found that, technically, it's the melody, it's the key.

PD: It's not just a note, but a collection of notes?

JJ: More the collection, the juxtaposition of notes side-by-side. I had an Alzheimer's patient who was in her 90s, and with just a few notes from me she sang Jesus Loves Me, word for word, which she learned when she was in Sunday school. She couldn't remember that her mother had died, but she could remember that song. Neurologically, I think it is the connection of the note with the word. So I find, in this profound effect music has, it's the notes, it's the melody, it's the harmonies, it's the words, and it's the associations we make with the music, all connected.

Often, though, the words don't have to be there for the

music to have an impact. My husband is from Istanbul, Turkey, and when we go there to visit, they always ask me to sing "that sad song." They don't know English, and when they say, "that sad song," they mean *Danny Boy*. They don't understand what the song is about, but they know it's sad.

PD: So they know it's sad from the minor chords?

JJ: It's not minor, Peter, it's D major! Very often the minor keys do create in us a sense of sadness, but this song is a case in point; it's just the music, it's not the words. Now, we can think of symphonic music that can create in us a sense of sadness or, very often, sadness and happiness together. I think of Beethoven's *Ode to Joy*, that creates in me a sense of joy and sadness at the same time. So music has that ability to address our opposite emotions, which can be very much present in palliative care.

PD: And it has a way to pierce through even a disease like Alzheimer's?

JJ: In that way it reaches everybody. Now, it is the music, it is the words, and it is the feeling that's created from this. I often get a sense of warmth, of comfort and strong emotions that are all elicited from the words and music together.

Music can take our woundedness, our pain, and our sorrows away, out of our soul, leaving us healed and whole and at peace, even for just a song. It's for the moment. But that's what palliative care is about – to give this person what comfort they can have at this moment in their lives.

PD: Was it Ian who was the country and western fan?

JJ: Yes, and I would sing his favorites to uplift his mood. Now, when I would come on the floor, he'd say, "Jenny's here! You go get your guitar, dear, and you come back, because we're going to sing a song!"

He told me he loved country and western and so I said, "How about The Crystal Chandelier, Ian?"

"You bet, I just love that."

So I'd start, "Ooooh, the crystal chandelier...," and I'd sing it with my country accent, my nose plugged and everything, and he would start to sing with me. He'd sing so loud that his roommate, who was almost deaf, could hear him. His roommate, who was a lot older and very quiet, was often just in the corner, hands crossed and head down. And when Ian and I would start to sing this, he'd look up and he'd smile. After that, I said, "Ian, let's sing something that Jack might know."

"You bet! Let's do that, dear."

And we sang, "Daisy, Daisy, give me your answer do..." Ian was singing in his loud, base voice. And Jack, this little man, was singing in a high tenor voice – this man who was almost deaf, who appeared quite lonely.

So we developed this group feeling of warmth, of sharing together. It alleviated his isolation, his loneliness, and he experienced an uplifting of his mood.

PD: Do you think there's a physical impact as well ?

JJ: Yes. I feel it's physiological, emotional, spiritual. Anthony Storr goes into depth talking about how music causes an increased arousal in those who are listening to it, almost whether we like it or not.

PD: I wonder if it's possible that, when the physical body is facing termination, maybe the mind seeks the familiar, and music is just a perfect vehicle for delivering the familiar.

JJ: Yes! And because a lot of the songs I use are familiar to the patient, there's a sense of comfort in just that familiarity. A comfort unto itself: "I know that song. That song reminds me of when I went to church, or when my dad sang that."

PD: Didn't Ian listen to a tape of your music the night he was dying?

JJ: Yes he did.

I was told that the night he died he played my tape and it brought him a sense of comfort. He called his wife, he told her he loved her. He was at peace with himself, and the music brought him so much joy.

One day, we were singing our duets together, and he said, "Jenny, next time you come, I'm getting a blank tape and we're going to tape our duets and I can't wait!" And I was excited, I was looking forward to it too. But the next week Ian was gone. He had died. So I missed that opportunity.

For me, it was a sadness, because I had lost this friend, this musical fun that we had together. But when the nurse told me that he had played my music, I felt that, in a sense, I had a presence with him indirectly.

PD: I was going to say you were a partner on that journey.

JJ: Yes. And that's special. It is also powerful. Because it's so powerful, I have to be careful. I could misuse it.

PD: In what way?

JJ: If I offer *Abide With Me*, or sing it, when the patient is not ready for it, that can hurt them. That's why I always ask for their preferences. What do you like? What style of music do you like? What shouldn't I sing? And they will tell me.

PD: I couldn't see the face of the first patient you were singing *Amazing Grace* to this afternoon. Was there a reaction at all, could you sense that you were touching her?

JJ: I sensed some touching. I think she was in a coma, Peter. I find that with patients who are in a coma, they respond on a different level and often it's not a physical response that you can see. Maybe their breathing calms. I saw her eyes look at me for a slight second.

PD: The family obviously reacted with some emotion and it was...

JJ: At that stage, Peter, I do address my music toward the family. I direct my singing to her, but I say to them, "Listen to the words and the meaning that they have, that they can give to you." In that way, I want them to take in the music and the comfort it can give them. When the person is that close to death, I often direct my therapy to the family.

PD: The music must change, the requests must change for you as the illness progresses?

JJ: They do. I'm very sensitive, at the beginning, when I meet a patient. I do not offer songs such as *Abide With Me*, or *Amazing Grace*, or *Danny Boy*. I've learned that these songs are more difficult, patients are not ready to hear them, they're not ready to accept the song or the words. Very often, the family members will say, "Do not sing *Danny Boy*, do not sing *Abide With Me*." I'm very sensitive to that, so of course I don't.

PD: Because the family isn't ready or the patient isn't ready to hear that, do you think?

JJ: It's usually the family, most often it's the family that's not ready.

PD: Who don't want to face...

JJ: They don't want to hear it.

Now, I worked with one couple and a lot of my work with this couple involved reminiscing. That's one of my main goals – reminiscing, bringing back fond memories, reinforcing self-identity, who they've been, talking about when they were married. And so with this one couple, we talked about when they courted. One day, I went in with the theme of love and I sang just love songs. And when I sang, "Let me call you sweetheart, I'm in love with you...," Les sang along with me, he looked at his wife, he blew her kisses, he held her hand.

They experienced the sense of love and relationship they had because after each song I said, "Tell me about when you first dated," and they were thrilled to recount that whole memory with me.

Les's wife was, I think, pushing away the fact that he was going to die and not thinking about the issues related to that. So she would say to me, "No, I don't want to hear *Danny Boy*, I don't want to hear *Amazing Grace*."

After five or six weeks, I decided I was going to sing some hymns. Obviously, if they were atheist, I wouldn't do that, but I knew they were members of the United Church, so I brought those songs with the purpose of having her face her emotions. As I sang *Amazing Grace*, she cried for the first time.

Now I would never do that in the first couple of sessions, because I haven't developed a relationship or a trust yet. But I knew, by the fifth or sixth visit, that I had her trust; she knew I wasn't going to do anything against her emotions and feelings. But I wanted to bring this about, this facing of emotions, the fact that Les was going to die soon.

I say now that, when people cry, they are healing tears, they are tears that have to come out at some point, and the sooner they come out, maybe the better.

PD: Why is it important for them to come out? In a healing sense, what's your understanding of what that process allows to happen?

JJ: Well, I think the tears show them that this is happening: "I have to deal with it. These are my feelings deep within me. I cannot reject them or ignore them anymore." When you're crying, you can't ignore that you're crying. When she's at home and doing all her cleaning work, she can ignore her feelings. But with a song such as *Amazing Grace*, or later I sang *Danny Boy*, she can't turn her ears off. So she's hearing the music, and it can't help but affect her, it penetrates her soul.

I don't think anyone can put a wall up toward music. We can't stop it from affecting us. So it affected her. It made her cry. It made her face reality. It was at that point, I think, that she started her grief process. The tears and the music stimulated that.

PD: It must change your mind about "wellness," because people aren't getting better here. I wonder how you see healing now?

JJ: I see healing on this floor in a spiritual sense, in a psychological sense. People may feel more at peace. Spiritually, they may feel more ready after they hear *The Lord is My Shepherd*.

PD: What's the reception like when you first meet.

JJ: It's hard. I find that I'm often greeted with skepticism. They don't know what I'm there to offer. So I'm very sensitive to their feelings.

PD: What do you say? What do you say that you want to do when you walk into a room like that?

JJ: I say, "Can I offer you some music? Is there some music that has had meaning in your life that I can share with you? Would you like to have a visit? I'll just sing some quiet songs and then go."

Or the nurse might go in for me and say, "Would you like to have music." Now that's a nice interaction and introduction because they know the nurse, they trust the nurse, and the nurse is saying, "Oh just listen to this dear girl sing a song for you."

But I'm very soft, gentle, not pushy in any way, and if they say "no," that's fine.

Very often, they'll hear me in another room and then the next week say, "Hey, do you want to come and sing for me now." So it's a very gentle, soft approach. I'm very accepting of their desires and needs.

PD: It's true that our lives are sometimes defined by music. The music around the war was, and still is, intoxicating for people who went through that. Music defines chapters of your life.

JJ: That's how I can encourage reminiscences. I'll find songs that had meaning in their childhood, in their teen years, when they married. I often ask what the song was at their wedding. I had one gentleman who wanted to hear me sing *Ave Maria* every week and he reminisced about his wedding. He told me every detail of his wedding after I sang that song and it...

PD: Opened up the floodgates. When did you realize the power of music?

JJ: I think it has struck me here, working with palliative care people who are facing the end of their life – that's profound in itself. And I have seen the music touch people in such profound ways here. Now, when I work with little children and I sing *Baa Baa Black Sheep*, well they're so excited and I see the energy that it brings them and the happiness and the pure pleasure. But here it's on a different level. I think once I really got started working here, I found it to be profound in its effect. When I was studying, I never got this opportunity. So it's come to me since I've been a music therapist for a couple of years and I've been with patients.

PD: So it's growing, the more you work the more you see.

JJ: And I think I'm a more effective music therapist because I can be more sensitive to the songs, to the patients, and to how to work with them.

PD: Does it ever not work? Have you ever had anyone for whom it just didn't strike a chord?

JJ: I have had patients tell me they don't want music, they don't particularly like it. But for all the others who say, "Yes, come and sing with me," I have had some reaction and from all different levels.

PD: It must be very sad to have friends leaving you all the time?

JJ: It is, but I think you adjust because you really have no choice. Often, when you come back, there's someone else in that bed, there is a family with new needs that you have to pick up and address right away.

What's special, though, is that I have all the memories: of Les, of Ian, of Margaret. Of this one woman who just loved religious music and, for me, when I arrived on the floor, she got out her hymnal. She said to the nurse, "You come and have a singalong with me." She had everyone in her room. We would have a hymn sing. She would look at me and say, "Jenny, I feel through your music that I'm in touch with God." It was so spiritually important and valued for her.

I think for the family today to hear *Amazing Grace*, *The Lord Is My Shepherd*, it brought them a spiritual comfort, they want to know that their loved one is going to go to heaven.

PD: And words alone don't do it.

JJ: I don't think they do it nearly as strongly as when they are combined with the music.

I also use music to induce relaxation and reduce the

perception of pain. A lot of the patients here are in pain. I will sing to them with the goal of taking their mind off the pain in their leg, say, and focusing it on the words or the melody. And for that moment, they often don't feel pain. One gentleman here was experiencing severe pain, and I would use the music to distract his thoughts away from the pain. For the moment of the song, he'd look at me and listen to the music. He'd think of the songs. His daughter wrote a letter saying, "Jenny, you took my dad away from his pain to a world without pain." I know it was not for the entire day, but for a moment.

PD: Tell me about Bobby who only responded to music.

JJ: Bob lives in a group home. Usually, he is in the kitchen, rocking and grunting. I say, "Bob, it's time for music," and he looks up, he becomes alive, and he comes into the living room. I give him a drum and he beats with perfect rhythm and we sing our Indian song, My *Paddle's Keen and Bright*.

Then I sing, "Bob and Jenny are playing the drum..." to the same tune and he will continue singing it without me. I was gone for six months on maternity leave and the first session that we had together when I got back, he sang that like he had never forgotten a thing. The connection with music is so...

PD: Profound.

JJ: And successful. He became alive, he became appropriate in his social interactions, in the way he talked. He doesn't talk a lot. His favorite song is *Working on the Railroad*. So, as an activity, I'll sing, "I've been working on the...," and he'll sing, "railroad." I'll continue, "All the live long...," and he'll respond with, "day." So he will give what he can from that song. I think he experiences so much success that he feels good. It increases his self-esteem, he smiles, he laughs. It's so wonderful to see that transformation. One moment he's rocking and grunting, the next he's smiling, laughing, singing and playing a drum.

PD: And how do you feel at that point? Responsible? Powerful?

JJ: I feel his excitement because when he's laughing, it makes me want to laugh too. I have a bit of a high that I've shared the music and that I've made him feel that success and that happiness. That's what makes my work so rewarding, because I have these responses all the time.

PD: What's the reaction of health care professionals on a floor like this? How do they regard you and what you do?

JJ: At first I think there was skepticism because it was unknown. What's music therapy? They didn't know about it so I had to show them. I had to demonstrate. I volunteered for about eight months to show this is what music therapy is all about.

Now I have the most wonderful trust and relationships with the nurses and the doctor. When I come in, they say, "Oh, Jenny, I know just the person for you to see and, by the way, they're Irish and, by the way, they're Christian. And they told me this is their favorite song." Now I'm part of the team, a multi-disciplinary team. I can be included and I can give to them information from my experiences.

You see, that story I told you about the father and his two sons, where I sang, "I love you, you love me..." Well, this man was so warm and gentle and sweet with me. He'd say things such as, "Jenny, music is like a warm blanket to me. Thank you for the music, it means so much to me." When I told that to a nurse, she was shocked. Her mouth dropped open and she said, "He said what? He did what? He just swears at us. He throws his juice at us and he'll tell us to get the hell out of here and stop coming in. He doesn't want to see us." I was shocked because I hadn't experienced that.

PD: You'd seen the other side.

JJ: I'd seen the other side because of the positive effect the music had. Now because I offered that story, it brought something new to the team and they realized the music is effective and it works for this gentleman.

Often, I'll try to get in a team meeting and share with the team what experiences and reactions I've had with the patients. One individual was very depressed and the nurses and doctors always talked about how depressed this person was. I explained that during my visits, I'd see not so much a depression but a reaction, a positiveness, an interest.

PD: It's almost as if the music allows them to be human, to open up.

JJ: It does.

PD: It opens up avenues for them that maybe otherwise they don't feel comfortable with?

JJ: That's right. I'm not related to their pain, whereas maybe the nurses and doctors are because they have to give the medication. They have to go in and say, "We have to turn you now," and all those things. But I can get another side from a patient and I think that's so important in this situation.

PD: Does it help you? Are you a different person after spending three hours on this floor?

JJ: I always go home feeling rewarded. I'm always saying to my husband how much I love my work. It means so much to me and I see that it has meaning to the people I work with. I see the joy I bring to children, I see the excitement and the motivation with handicapped adults, and here, I see the peace and comfort that I can give patients and family members.

One day I was in the nurses' center and one of them said, "Jenny, would you sing us a song, just for us." I started with *Blowing in the Wind* and they took in that music like vitamins for the soul. The next week when I came in, the one nurse said, "Jen, I went home that night and I felt lighter. And I thought, 'What happened,' and boom it hit me, the music!" It was healing and comforting to her.

Very often I'm in a situation where I'm singing to a patient and a nurse is there and, after six weeks, they've developed a relationship too. They'll often hold the patient's hand while I'm singing a song and be in that atmosphere and that warmth.

PD: How far do you think music therapy can go? What are the possibilities?

JJ: They are numerous. Music therapy was first introduced in psychiatric hospitals and there is an amazing healing and therapy that is done through the music. Today it is offered in hospitals, prisons, schools, nursing homes, group homes. It is successful with so many special populations.

I'm working with an autistic girl right now and we're getting at her emotions. She doesn't know what happy, sad, and mad are. So we're improvising these emotions on the piano. She's experiencing mad through the music and she loves it. Instead of screaming, she's playing the piano in a mad way. At the time we were doing a sad song, this girl's grandma died and she experienced sadness, but she seemed to grasp it, understand it more, through the music. Music does make the person more whole.

PD: I guess what I meant by the possibilities is that I think we only understand a fraction of how our bodies and minds work, and if we ever did really honor music for the role that it could play...

JJ: Or the arts in general...

PD: Or the arts in general, we'd probably stop taking so many drugs, we'd stop the way we've been practicing medicine.

JJ: And I think we are turning to the alternative approaches. It's not just medical anymore. And that's why I'm so accepted here in palliative care, because the cure is no longer the goal. These people are dying and so what better time to offer something different, to bring in the arts, to bring in music.

Art therapy, dance therapy, the creative art therapies, I think, should find a lot more acceptance in the 21st century. Certainly, if we accepted music and art in our lives more, I think everyone would be healthier.

Chapter 3
NIGHTTIME WHISPERS

The Mystery of Healing Dreams

Jim & Donna Sinclair

☙

ॐ

**"The dream is a little hidden door in the innermost and
most secret recesses of the psyche, opening into the
cosmic night..." – Carl Jung**

*Carl Jung, of course, is the great contemporary guide to our
dreams and while they play a significant role in the Christian
experience, Jung's suggestion that they open a door to a vast and
dark richness seems a good first step in explaining the intense
human curiosity and passion for the subject.*

*The power of image in our lives is incontestable and so it
seems logical that those which bubble up to the surface of our
consciousness in our sleep exert a powerful influence on our health
and well-being, if we honor and respect their presence. While
dreaming comes naturally to all of us, not everyone knows how
to "read" them. It takes a little work to understand the language
of these nighttime whispers and that's where people such as Jim
and Donna Sinclair can help. Both have years of interest and
experience in dream work.*

*Jim is a United Church minister and Donna is a writer. They
live in North Bay, Ontario, and once a month, they welcome
people to the church for a dream workshop.*

ॐ

PD: Do you remember when you first realized that dreams could be significant?

JS: We were intrigued. As a couple, we had good friends in Quebec – a colleague and his partner. We got together at that time, I think it was every Sunday night.

DS: Yes. We all had little kids and we were just exhausted, but we'd get together and talk about dreams. And we could hardly keep our eyes open!

PD: So how did that start? Was it your idea, do you remember?

DS: Actually it was our friends' idea. They were heavily into Jung and started to talk with us about it. I think because we were good friends, we trusted this odd stuff and got into it.

PD: Did it seem "odd" to you at first?

DS: It's so hard to remember back then. No, speaking for myself. My background was English literature and it kind of felt like a poem.

JS: It did for me at first. I can remember we went for several years to Five Oaks, the United Church center in Paris, Ontario, and there was a gentleman there named Russ Becker, who had held the chair in pastoral theology at Yale.

During the Vietnam war, he decided that he needed to do something that would really revitalize the church. He left the chair and went back into the pastorate and became heavily involved in dream work after spending a year in

Switzerland at the Jungian Institute. He then ran this dream group at Five Oaks for several years.

PD: So he really made it, I don't know if "legitimate" is the right word, but it seemed that it could be a serious part of your ministry?

JS: Yes, and part of my life. I think it was the first time we went. There were only 18 there at the time – a very disparate group of people. We began to work on a dream that I had had and I can remember, as we worked on the dream, these "Aha!" responses. I was quite surprised and I felt quite helped by what we did. I never felt like a "new convert" or anything, but my background is in clinical therapy and I found this to be very helpful.

PD: Can I go back for a second to those Sunday night sessions in the Eastern Townships. Donna, you said they were intriguing. What were they like? What happened at them?

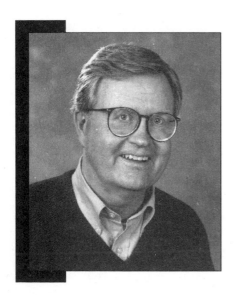

DS: There was just the four of us. We'd have supper together, put the kids to bed, and then we'd all sit around and share dreams and usually take turns.

PD: Had you written them down?

DS: Yea. That's fairly important because you lose them

pretty fast. It was really like giving each other a little en-capsulated glimpse of what the week had been like, in terms of dreams.

PD: And then the group would try to interpret them?

DS: Yes, and there was a lot of trust, of course, amongst the four of us.

PD: There'd have to be, I guess.

JS: We did that for a couple of years.

PD: I know it's difficult to look back through all the years of experience you have now, but did you think, back then, that dreams did, in fact, have a healing quality to them?

DS: I probably wouldn't have used the word "healing" at that point. I don't think my definition of healing was as broad as it is now. I think I just felt that this was expanding my life. This was making me more aware of a whole lot of things – of who I was. But I wouldn't have used the word healing.

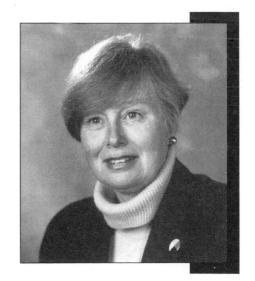

PD: Jim?

JS: I can remember, at the time, I said, "This is church for me." I had a four-point pastoral charge and we loved that congregation. But for me, anyway, worship was, in large measure, fairly task-oriented.

I was responsible for many of the things that happened, and so by Sunday evening I was really tired, I needed to be soothed.

I would say now that there was certainly a therapeutic character and a healing quality, but, like Donna, I wouldn't have thought of it as healing *per se*.

PD: But you do now?

JS: Yes, very much so.

PD: Donna, what are the ingredients of healing? How would you define it now?

DS: Well, it's something that affects the spiritual, the emotional, the physical, and the mental. Actually, I don't think I'd separate those in any way. It's whatever helps a person live their life more fully, I guess.

If part of that includes moving from a state where you are unhappy or not functioning well to a state where you are happy or where the sky seems bluer, that's healing! And so that might mean that persistent pains here or there disappear. It might mean that.

PD: You know the word that keeps coming up is balance, that healing means to recover a balance that we lose somehow in our everyday life.

DS: That's actually a nice definition of what dreams do.

JS: Yes.

DS: Dreams are always aiming at a psychic balance and always trying to compensate for an overemphasis, perhaps, on the rational. Whatever way we tend to overbalance ourselves in the way we go through life, the dreams will try to correct.

JS: I agree. I think balance is a very important part of it. But I was also thinking that healing would include a sense of validation, of affirmation.

Another word that I would put into the definition would be "connection," that there is a sense that me is part of our. I'm part not just of something around me in this life, but I'm connected with meaning, with something beyond my own agenda, and I am important within that larger context.

PD: It certainly seems that we are feeling disconnected, that more and more people are feeling they haven't got a place in the universe. What I wonder about sometimes is whether that's always been the case, or is there something now, as we approach the 21st century, that is highlighting that sense of being alone?

JS: Well, that's one of the great religious motifs – alienation. Another word for me would be brokenness. That's why connectedness is important to me within a definition of healing. Healing might involve the brokenness within our body, but it might also be the brokenness with other individuals.

Dreams might be one vehicle for people who have yet to find something helpful, to feel more connected with their spirituality.

PD: And traditional methods may not have appealed to them or they may not be open to them?

JS: That's right. One of the things we've experienced as United Church folks is that we have a lot of people who attend who have either another religious affiliation or who have none. So for some people, there is an active connection with the church. But I would say the norm would be, in the groups we've had every year, people who have a deep spiritual dimension to their character or journey and this seems to be another way of getting them going. And for some of them, it's quite fulfilling.

PD: So do you think that sense of being alone, of not being connected, is larger now than it has been in the past? Donna?

DS: It's one of those questions that unleashes a volcano! We see it around us, politically, in Ontario, and globally – this increasing sense that human beings are disparate units that can be moved around like little building blocks. There's no sense of the connectedness of society. Society is just a bunch of mechanistic blocks that you can do with as you will without worrying about the links and connections between them or about what the fabric of all those woven interconnections might be.

So, if for no other reason than that our culture seems to be going in the opposite direction of that sense of compensation or of balance, I think people will be yearning for anything that will help them connect with each other or with the warring parts of themselves.

PD: So in that context, how do dreams help people reconnect with themselves or with other people?

DS: I think dreams come from a very deep and very personal part of ourselves. So when we dredge that up and begin to share it – whether or not people can interpret it or respond to it – we are offering a part of ourselves. People treat that with enormous respect. So, in that sense, it is a connection.

But then you get the response! When people begin to come back and say, "You know, I see this," or "This makes me feel like this," or "I read a poem where that particular object seemed to mean this," they're all working collectively on this very precious part of one person's self. That's very intimate.

PD: And powerful.

DS: Oh yes. It's like being present at the creation sometimes! You have the sense of wanting to take off your shoes because this is holy ground.

JS: One of the principles that we've worked on in dream interpretation is that every element within the dream – whether it's a person or otherwise – is a part of ourselves. Or at least, we try to explore what that element would mean if we related it to ourselves.

PD: It's interesting that dreams can reveal the pressures that you may not be aware of, on sort of a daily basis, but that are weighing heavily on you.

JS: Yes. And what about the dreams of people in a war zone or the dreaming of people in poverty? One of my hunches is that a lot of people, who are not sleeping or eating properly, are losing their dreams. Unless there is a context in which their dreams can be valued and validated, the dreams are not the tools they might be otherwise.

PD: In a general way, can you describe what happens at your sessions and what some of the wounds are that you see being healed by the validation of people's dreams?

DS: Well, we gather once a month as a large group. We visit for a while, have coffee, and then we might talk for half an hour about something someone has read or about a question someone has. It used to be, when we first started the monthly meetings, that Jim and I would do a lot of theory. We don't anymore because a lot of these people know more about dreams than we do and are studying really hard. So we just share knowledge or ideas.

JS: To find a safe place where you feel secure, even with people you've never met before, is very healing.

It has that flavor of being on a plane with a stranger and you discover you've said things that you've never said to anybody else! But it's not that we're never going to meet these people again – we'll see each other at the next dream group. Although that may be the only time during the week we see each other. That's actually one of the remarkable things about our group – for the most part we only see each other at the group. Most are not congregational members, although some are.

DS: There may be 20 or 30 people for the large group, so then we break into small groups of four or five, some of which are fairly permanent. The same four or five people will meet all the time and they develop a remarkable ability to work very intimately on each other's dreams. And then other groups, particularly if they're new people, will be more fluid. Jim and I will usually go off with people who have never been to a dream group before. We go into separate corners of the church so that every small group has their own space. There's some fairly intensive work that goes on in the groups.

JS: A lot of people are sustained by this and it is a surprise to me from time to time. Often, to be very frank, we get to Friday night, when there is going to be a dream group, and we're exhausted. And we think "Whoa," we've made the commitment. And yet when we go there we get energized.

We discover there are people there who remind us by their own behavior that they need their dreams.

DS: The usual pattern is that people take turns reading their dreams. They use a variety of methods in the group to, first, honor the dream, and then to come to some ideas about what the dream might be trying to say.

So they might do active imagining or amplification or free association. People will say, "Gee, this makes me think of..." And then they'll go on from there, until the dreamer, who's always in charge and who always "owns" the dream, says, "Well, thank you." Then they go on to the next person's dream.

People are quite careful of one another, both in the sense of not jumping in with an interpretation before a person's ready to hear it, but also in terms of not hogging the whole evening! There's quite an elaborate but unconscious etiquette, I think, around the dreams.

PD: That shows a respect for the power of them, I think.

JS: Very much so.

PD: Nobody wants to be too quick to judge, understanding that it comes from a place that is greater than everybody in the group, I suppose.

DS: Yes. And then we all go home. The small groups break up at various times and the last one out does the dishes!

PD: Are there themes that keep arising, that people are troubled by?

JS: Certainly. It's often around the question of intimacy, and I don't mean sexual relationships, although that occasionally comes up.

That's always very scary for people, when the issue of sexual relationships comes up. It's a teachable moment for us: how are we going to handle that kind of material if anybody chooses to present it?

But more often, it's people struggling with what it means to get close to "whatever." Now that could be a person, or it could be something within themselves that's happening and that they haven't really been able to come to grips with.

For some people, the issue is what it would mean to be closer to, I would say "God," but some of them don't think in those terms. It's certainly a higher power – meaning beyond their own situation. And I think that's where the context, the fact that we meet in a church, often fosters or at least supports people in the very thing that they're seeking.

Currently, we also see people expressing the corporate

anxiety of the day. We've had people struggling to discern their future direction, both vocationally and otherwise.

We also spend time looking at the ethical dimension of what it means to handle material like this: how to be present when it's shared, how to honor and respect it when it's offered, and then how to let go of it so that it only leaves the room through the person who has offered it in the first place.

Before we got into the monthly stuff, we used to do a weekend in the fall and a weekend in the spring. We would have people come to those events who would change their vocation as the result of some things that they released.

I would say now, looking back, that it wasn't the event that prompted it, it was that the event was one of a series of things in their discernment process. But in those cases, they had crystallized some things and they were trying them out loud, both to themselves and to other people.

DS: I see people working on issues from childhood, childhood pain which all of us have, and going back and revisiting that in the safety of the group and doing some healing.

Women, I think, are probably hyperalert to this. So they work on women's issues – issues of dependence and independence. And they struggle to discern how they can be a woman in today's world. Also, people come with broken relationships that they need to talk through.

And there's another interesting issue that I was thinking of while Jim was talking. We have a lot of artists, people whose lives are wrapped up in producing art. Somehow they've all kind of moved in. I think we often see the kind of issues that creative people have to struggle with when they face the world: the meaning of their art, how people receive it, what happens when a person has all their antennae up and is very sensitive and open and vulnerable – and I think an artist is all those things – how do they make their way through life? That, in a way, is a wounding.

PD: I don't know if there's an answer to this, but does it matter to you what the source of the dream is, and is it important to know where it comes from?

JS: I think it's a critical question. As the groups work with individuals on their dreams, you'll see different levels. People can understand a dream on one level, or they can understand it on another level. And sometimes the dream, as Donna suggests, might well refer to a very early time in the person's life.

I'm just thinking of a woman who's had a series of broken relationships, who may suddenly come to an understanding of why she is having trouble with intimacy, and it's expressed not only in her most personal relationships but in many other ways as well.

But that gets into the question of how you define what a group like this provides, and whether or not it's actual therapy. We're always struggling with that in a way, with the potential of being seen as irresponsible and not professional. Are we ethical, skilled, and all of that sort of thing? I think those are questions that we struggle with and they're related to the very question that you're asking.

There is a point when you see where this dream could be coming from; we don't know for sure, so what do we do next? As responsible leaders, we are participants in a dynamic that has its own synergy. We certainly feel a responsibility for people not getting hurt by suddenly being given more than they can handle. The question becomes more critical, I think, the more pain people feel.

DS: I think part of what you're asking though, Peter, is whether they come from God or whether they come from inside ourselves?

PD: Yes. I guess whether people see it as a message as much as they see it as something in us. One of the things that has also been coming up is this idea that we are all healers ourselves, that we all have the capacity to heal. You see, I wonder if people want to believe these are messages from God?

DS: It's such an interesting question. I believe myself that they come from God.

JS: We've used as the title for our group "Dreams: God's Forgotten Language," which is the title of a book by John A. Sanford.

DS: I'm very conscious, though, that some of the people who come to the group have not had happy experiences with church. They may have had to drag themselves over the threshold of this building. So I tend to be a little reluctant about pushing that too hard. Jim's more comfortable with it and it rests better with him, partly because of his role.

PD: Right.

DS: I think the group would be clear that we believe that this is God talk that we're about, but there's certainly no need for everyone to subscribe to that. If they would prefer to believe that it originates somewhere within themselves, in some kind of recess of their unconscious that has no connection with God, I think that would be okay.

JS: It certainly isn't a proselytizing sort of thing and I can't remember anybody over the years making an effort to do that. But we've certainly had people who, I think, see the insights that come to them as coming from God.

And yet we have looked at it within the context of a Jungian framework, so when people find the jester or the wise old woman, or some of these archetypal images within their dreams, some people may leave it at that. They may see it simply as part of the collective unconscious which has been well-documented, in many ways, by people such as Jung and others.

But other people may then choose to go beyond that and say, "Well, my way of understanding this would be that it is from God and it is part of my spiritual discernment." We have encouraged people – as part of the discipline of looking at dreams – to ask questions of their dreams, to say, "Well okay, maybe that's what this dream is." It's not to offer an answer, but to help you shape the right question for the days yet to come.

We've had people affirm that they go to bed at night and ask a question of their dreams and feel that they've furthered the endeavor by the kind of things that actually occur the next time around.

PD: But even staying in touch with yourself or whatever power there is, can help you to avoid becoming disconnected.

JS: That makes me think of when we lived in Cowansville. I would refer couples for marriage counseling to people in Montreal. Inevitably, I would hear back, both from the couple and from the counselor, what a wonderful evening they had had, even when they'd gone to discuss significant areas of conflict.

The counselor's comment was that, on occasion, the drive to Montreal – and sometimes the couple would stay for supper or to see a show – was more helpful than the actual work that they were attempting to do in the counseling.

PD: It's always struck me as being a bit like telling ghost stories. People love sitting around talking about their dreams. It's true isn't it that there is something communal about sharing those whispers?

JS: Very much so.

DS: It's a mystery, it's very mysterious.

PD: But if it's true that the dialogue between our brain and our body is in a language of images, then it seems to me the healing potential of dreams must be enormous.

JS: Well, if you see that image in other contexts, if you see it acted out by other people, if you recognize it in literature – I'm thinking of all that life script stuff where a therapist tries to help a person name the script that they are living – and if you find, within a process like that, images that echo with what you've been dreaming about and you can transfer that into your behavior, or your prayer life, or your worship life, or your art, that's certainly going to be efficacious.

PD: Something very powerful happens when we close our eyes and let go of this world.

DS: Yes.

JS: It's allowing for the irrational. We're dealing with people who are very much of a culture that can compartmentalize. Yes, we want and need to get the deficit down, but I think some would find it very difficult to come to grips with the fact that 100,000 single mothers and their children have been dislocated in Toronto and have moved into often inadequate housing as a result. Some can't see the connection.

PD: Or refuse to see it. Have either of you ever had a dream that has really made a difference in your life?

JS: I find that if I come up with dreams in which there is flying or in which I'm flying, I know now, from past experience, that I am probably out of control.

Now, I have to examine each dream in and of itself, but typically, those dreams come to me when I am stretched to the limit and I probably haven't been taking very good care of myself.

PD: Emotionally and physically out of control?

JS: In every respect. I'm a struggling workaholic and sometimes I handle that better than other times. But I know that my effectiveness and my health is compromised, or at least I know when I get a dream like that, so the first thing I've got to do is stop. And I ask myself, "Am I in a very balanced situation at the moment?"

So that's one of the things dreams offer me. I've come to claim that as one of its meanings. I have to be careful that it doesn't automatically mean that, but that's my first response.

PD: Sometimes they don't mean anything, is that possible?

JS: Yes. That's the other thing we've talked about in our group. Sometimes a dream is simply a gift in and of itself and it may just be taken for what it is.

Some of these dreams, especially the ones that are very affirming, need to be held up like fine china and simply enjoyed for what they are. They may not be all that practical.

PD: Donna, have you gained any sort of personal insight through your dreams?

DS: Oh yes, some similar to Jim. I had one in particular that I love. I was trying to squeeze a whole bunch of children, about 20, into a Volkswagen to get to a play. And when I worked on it, the dream seemed to be saying, "You've got so many interesting, creative projects on the go that you can't get your act together!" Dreams will often come along and charge me with overdoing it.

I had a whole series in which the dreams seemed to be saying, "You know, you're being a little too rigid with your children, particularly the oldest one, and you should let up." This was when he was about six. And I did! And we've had really quite a remarkably fine relationship ever since.

One of the things that goes on in our house now is that our youngest daughter, who is 16, will bring all her friends home and sometimes they'll all charge into my study and sit down and say, "So-and-so has had a dream!" This may be *apropos* of nothing, but dreams for that little group of adolescents are not scary things. They just know that they're things you talk about.

PD: Well maybe that is *apropos* of healing, though. We live in a culture that is so violent these days that a dream is such a gentle whisper. I was reassured by the idea that teenagers would use their imagination or be excited by it. There's nothing aggressive about the process.

JS: Well, there is the nightmare material. However, people often discover that the nightmare which seems so debilitating turns out to be an affirmation or validation in another guise. It is a dream that comes when they are ignoring what they need. The dream takes a form that grabs them by the shoulders and says, "Look! Pay attention!"

DS: And when we allow ourselves to go into the dark like that, to walk into the mystery holding hands with each other, that is just so remarkable and healing in itself.

Chapter 4

HEART CONNECTIONS

The Healing Prayer of *Wayne Irwin*
& Flora Litt

As the snow melted and the earth was born again in the early spring of 1983, a new idea sprouted for Wayne Irwin's United Church congregation. He had tended the ground well, carefully considering the congregation's comfort and acceptance level. And so it was that 13 years ago, he decided the time was right to demonstrate a healing service in his church.

The use of prayer and the laying on of hands in a healing way is as old as the world itself and has played a role of varying importance in many traditions and belief systems through the ages. The cultural context, like the warming soil of spring, has much to do with how this practice grows. In North America, we know in our hearts the value of touch, but, too often, we don't welcome the mystery of our lives, and we allow our heads to lead us to demand scientific proof, as if, magically, that held all life's answers.

Clearly, all the wizardry and high-tech medical equipment has its place, but something invaluable is lost when we ignore the healing potential of prayer and the simple human acts of caring and touching and loving. Wayne Irwin and his colleague Flora Litt work at proving that every day.

PD: How did you come to connect healing with prayer?

FL: For me personally, it's always been an interest and an awareness that we can be channels of healing for other people.

In connection with the church, many years ago (13 since we held our first healing service) I was a member of the Christian development committee of the Halton Presbytery of the Hamilton Conference and at that time we organized a presbytery healing service. It was the first time that I laid hands on anyone for healing in a public way. We all smooth a brow, or put an arm around someone and send love and compassion and healing energy towards another without having to have any formal prayer language around it. But this was the first time, for me, that it had any formal church language around it. Although I've been in the church all my life, the church's ministry had not in my experience included healing in any overt way, other than the healing potential of confession and communion in worship.

PD: It was just assumed, I suppose.

FL: Well, we've always known that our Christian faith is healing.

PD: Wayne, the same for you?

WI: Yes, I think so. I grew up inside the church and it was part of the teaching that you could pray and intercede for somebody. But in terms of whether or not something happened as a result, there was a period in my life when I really wondered whether this was all just words we were saying or wishful thinking or what was going on. There were certainly times I wondered if, when we prayed for the well-being of things in South Africa for example, anything really happened there. I came through all of that, but it was because of others.

There was another United Church minister who was doing services of healing and I got involved in finding out what he was doing. It seemed foreign to our tradition.

It was partly because of my interest in physics. I said to myself, "Okay, we're putting hands on people, what's going on when we do that?" I wasn't prepared to involve people in the congregation until I could provide for them some kind of articulate expression of what was happening in the laying on of hands. There's a passage in the book of James that says that, when someone is sick, call for the elders and lay on hands, pray for them, and they will be healed. That was an intriguing passage. What did that mean? So that was in the mix of all of this. It was something that I was feeling drawn to myself.

However, I also had a sense that this was more commonplace in some other traditions, but that in ours it didn't seem

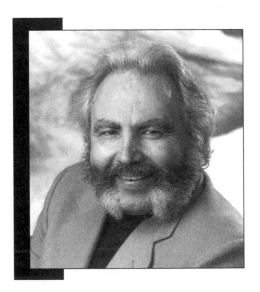

to be common. I've learned since then that it's in our background too. Wesley was much involved in healing – in the Methodist tradition – but I didn't know that at the time. I was aware that it was not just certain people who could do this. If healing was valid, it had to be something anybody could do. Those of us in the United

Church had to find out how this worked for us, as opposed to the spectacular ministry that we saw on television, some of which was off-putting for many people in our tradition.

PD: So tell me exactly what you do. What's involved?

FL: We have regular healing services and we've endeavored to come down the middle of the denomination in terms of style and of service format, and so we conduct them in the context of communion. It's very quiet and orderly. People come forward during the communion service. We have two healing rails, just small kneelers that we use, or a chair, or a person can stand. We're not hung up on how they receive; we do whatever is physically and emotionally comfortable for them. But they receive communion and then, if they wish to have prayer for themselves or for another person, they simply remain. There is a prayer team made up of two persons at each station, at each kneeler or chair. They lay hands on and pray. The prayer teams are comprised of both clergy and lay people because we believe in the concept of mutuality in ministry.

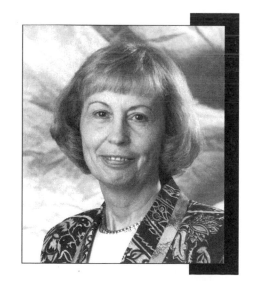

WI: It's not the bailiwick of only those in the Order of Ministry to anoint and lay on hands. Anyone can do this. Anyone can participate.

FL: And as for those who remain, sometimes they tell

us what they would like prayer for and sometimes not.

PD: How long does this take?

FL: We usually lay on hands and leave them where we put them – it may be a hand on a shoulder or head or it may be above the body in the same area – and we pray aloud, not because we have to, but because the person often feels better hearing words. Their belovedness is affirmed, their Divine connection is affirmed, and we hold up what we believe together. The length of time involved in that may be 30 seconds or two or three minutes. It's not long.

Now Therapeutic Touch is something a little different and is not something we do during a worship service. It is a treatment which involves an assessment of the energy field, an unruffling or clearing of the energy field, a redistribution of energy or a balancing of the field, and finally, a stabilizing of the field. So that is a certain process that may take 20 or 25 minutes from beginning to end.

PD: For someone who may not be familiar with that concept of the energy field of an individual, can you explain what you're doing and where your hands are going and why?

WI: The research that's been done on this is really the research for Therapeutic Touch. The primary scientist involved with this is Janet Quinn, who's an R.N. and Ph.D. in Boulder, Colorado. She worked back in the early 1980s on experiments using Therapeutic Touch with post-operative patients who were suffering from anxiety. In an earlier experiment, hands had been laid on patients, with touching and stroking. Janet redid the process three inches off the body and discovered that there was exactly the same outcome, in terms of alleviation of anxiety, as when they touched the body.

That was the first piece of actual research with data that showed there was something going on that didn't require actual physical contact, that you could have the same outcome or even a better outcome if you worked in this region of the body.

PD: Three inches above the body.

WI: Yes, in that general area, although not always. These days, they work with burn patients 12 inches above the body – it just depends. But these were actual *bona fide* scientific pieces of work, demonstrating that there was something happening that had just been a matter of speculation before.

Now some of these things also came out of Chinese theories of how we function and out of Indian science as well – traditional forms of understanding the body that are different from our Western way. They describe things such as acupuncture, or work with the idea of meridians, the flow of chi or vital force in the body. In addition, there's the idea that there's electrical movement within our body, and, whenever there is electrical movement, there is a field of energy.

All of this combines to undergird the concept that there is not only the physical aspect to things, there's also the energy of it; there's more to us than what we can see with the eye. We don't stop where our skin stops. We experience that in terms of our being in someone else's space. You know how, if someone has their foot in the door and you move up close to them, they'll back up. People seem to have...

PD: A comfort zone.

WI: Yes. That's a way in which most people would understand that there is something there, but it's very subtle.

PD: And the concept of resonance is helpful here.

WI: That's the word that I use. Resonance is a word from physics. When an electric charge passes through a coil, it causes a magnetic field. And when you bring another coil into proximity with that field, it causes an electrical flow. That's how a rheostat or dimmer switch works. When the coils are oriented at 90 degrees, no current flows. When you put them parallel, energy flows. Even though there's no direct contact, the energy flows and therefore the lights get brighter as you bring the coils into alignment. That is resonance.

So what's going on when we come into each other's field, when we come into close proximity with the other, is that this bioenergy that is moving within us influences the other person's energy.

So if we're angry and scattered, we're going to transmit that. If you're talking on the telephone with someone who is depressed, in 20 minutes you're depressed. It's the energetic connection with the other person. So if you're not protecting yourself, then you can become depressed.

The same thing can happen with healing. I once laid hands on a person many years ago who had a terrific earache, and after I was finished, I had an earache. It wasn't my earache, but I was feeling it. And so I thought, I have to learn how to do this a little better.

FL: We learn how to keep the flow going in one direction.

PD: How do you do that?

FL: Well, first of all, by your own alignment.

WI: And by deciding it in your own mind.

FL: If I'm attuned to peace and love, this will be a more powerful energy than the distress.

WI: That's a meditative method in which you get yourself centered.

FL: And then we connect with the other person and assess their field. So there are ways not to let the negative energy back in.

WI: It involves the mind.

FL: But sometimes it happens anyway.

WI: And the person on the other end can block it all the same way, by the mind. The person can say, "I'm not going to let this happen," and that's sufficient for it not to happen. So thought can block thought. We've learned, subconsciously, ways of protecting ourselves as we go through life. We learn how to block many things because so much is coming at us all the time. And the most vulnerable are infants and pets, and so not surprisingly, Therapeutic Touch is more effective with infants and pets.

Therapeutic Touch all started with a chap named Oskar Estebany who was a Hungarian soldier. He found that when he was wiping down his horse at night, his horse was calm while the other ones weren't. He had a particular knack for this. A scientist in Montreal, Bernard Grad, did experiments with healing back in the 1960s with Estebany. They created wounds in mice and Estebany laid hands on some of them and not on others and watched the difference in wound healing. It was significant.

And two other persons – Dolores Krieger, a nursing instructor, and Dora Kunz, a clairvoyant – were at a workshop with Estebany and asked if anybody could do this, to which he replied "no." They said, "We don't believe you." And so they went away and learned how to do it and how to teach it. And that was the beginning of Therapeutic Touch. Anybody can learn how to do this.

FL: The power of the mind is phenomenal.

WI: Part of the challenge for me was to find a way to provide this benefit for ordinary church people, in our ordinary laid-back Canadian way, who do not respond to things that are spectacular or in forms that put them off. Our people in the United Church, in general, prefer a peaceful, quiet kind of approach. If some people prefer the other, they know where they can go for that. We're endeavoring to offer something for the United Church because it doesn't need to be devoid of the possibility of healing liturgy.

FL: So besides the healing prayer and laying on of hands that we offer during communion in our worship services, we also teach Therapeutic Touch as part of the Prayer Centre healing ministry.

The Lowville Prayer Centre is a ministry of The United Church of Canada now. It's an incorporated special ministry and so we have workshops and seminars and teaching events. Healing services are now taking place in a number of locations.

But before we were the Lowville Prayer Centre, Wayne was having regular healing services within his own congregation.

WI: But trying, all the while, to find a way to do it that would work for our people who were not Anglican, Roman Catholic, or Pentecostal. Our folks needed to have the opportunity to get freed up and to be able to care for one another in such ways, because it had been lost, for the most part, in our tradition.

PD: How did you that? How did you introduce it in a way that, in the end, was acceptable, that wasn't frightening or intimidating?

WI: It was through the presbytery event held in 1983. There were a number of us who organized this service in Applewood Church in Mississauga. About 400 people turned up. We held a regular service and invited people to come forward for the laying on of hands. So it was a liturgical action that took place. A couple of hundred people, Order of Ministry persons and others, came forward and received healing prayer.

It happened that I had arranged for my choir to be present so there were 15 or 20 persons from my congregation who observed that this thing wasn't "off the wall." It was then possible for me to say, "How be we try it once?"

We did it in May, on a Wednesday evening, and invited people to come and pay attention to the fact that this Divine Mystery we call God is able to "do stuff." That's what we need to notice!

PD: To notice that God can "do" as well as "be."

FL: That God is present and active and involved in our lives. But we have become so heavy in the United Church on the preaching and the social action – wonderful as those are – that we've almost forgotten what we are really able to do by connecting with the power of God that moves through us.

We are getting invitations, requests from across the country, to come and help and teach about the healing ministry and how it can be opened up within our United Church. We're doing workshops and seminars in several places across the country this year.

PD: What's behind that demand do you think?

FL: An awareness! We have always known in the church that we were to be a healing community. In this secular world, there are many self-help and healing groups, support groups and healing communities. But the church has tended to look at it solely in spiritual terms and has not moved necessarily in this particular way with it, as have the Roman Catholics and the Anglicans and the Order of St. Luke and so on.

There's a timeliness to the hour now. I really do believe that the Spirit is moving through the field of science and moving through complementary therapies. There is this movement in the world today because we have gone about as far as we can go with the "head" on our own, without an awareness of the Divine intermingled with all of life. People live in isolation and this is a way that helps us know we're all connected. We are one community on this planet.

PD: In the spiritual, or mental, or emotional areas, are there "dis-eases" you're discovering again and again?

FL: Very often there's a spiritual ingredient that needs healing. It may be an issue of unforgiveness of self, or of anger against God. If the person is faith oriented, they may want to ask, "Where is God in an experience of abuse? Where is God in this healing process? Who am I as a spirit being, and what is the meaning of my life?" Those are the questions that ultimately a person has to address to stay whole, to bring their life into health and balance.

PD: There are an awful lot of us walking around who are not sure of where we fit in the universe.

FL: We ask: "Who am I? Why am I here?" We all need to discover that we are here to learn something, to grow, to develop, to give something, to contribute to the world, and that we are eternal, that our spirit nature is eternal. Then we can find meaning and relationship.

PD: So as people come to these healing stations you mentioned earlier and they want help, you're sensing or addressing their energy field?

FL: Yes and no. Since Wayne and I are qualified teachers of Therapeutic Touch and because we teach it for use in pastoral ministry within the church, some of our prayer team may be more aware of energy fields and so on. But we don't run our hands all over the person's aura or through their field when they're at the front of the church. We simply place our hands in the area of the head or the shoulders or the heart. Very often, if there's emotional pain, we may place a hand front and back, knowing that there are certain energy centers in the body.

It just depends. If a person comes forward with an

earache, we may place our hands there, but we know that the symptom that is described may not be where you want to put your hands anyway. And it really doesn't matter because if we are attuned to spirit, if we're attuned ourselves to spirit-level energy, then we are not going to transmit our own emotional stuff, we're not going to be sending our own thought forms. We're simply going to be praying, believing that the energy that's flowing through us will be distributed in that person's field or aura wherever it is needed. Regardless of whether it's a physical, emotional, or spiritual problem, the energy will go to where the healing is needed and the movement will be toward balancing, toward wholeness.

PD: And it can be for someone other than who is there at the moment?

FL: Absolutely! We make the connection with that other person through the one who's naming, speaking, or even holding that one in their heart, because their mental field, their whole emotional being, is attuned to that person.

In the laying on of hands, we do not do any physical contact necessarily. We're very gentle and respectful with our hands. Most often, they will simply be placed two or three inches away from the person, knowing that makes just as great an impact if not an even greater one than the physical touch.

So there's not any great technique about it. It's more about the openness of the other, and the most important ingredient is the love that flows. There have been experiments done to show that the effect of words, or no words, without compassion is so much less.

WI: There's an organization in Boulder Creek, California, called the HeartMath Institute that has been doing work on prayer and its effect on another person. They took EEG equipment and put it on a person who was praying and on the person who was being prayed for and began to monitor their brain waves. They observed that if the person doing the praying simply recited words, nothing happened in terms of what could be measured by this equipment. But they found that if the person doing the praying essentially concentrated on a loving intentionality for that other person, a caring deeply for that person's well-being that came from the heart, the brain waves of the person being prayed for began to entrain with the brain waves of the person praying, and the "spikes" on the two EEG readouts lined up exactly.

That kind of data was pretty astonishing because it showed that one person can have an effect on the physiology of another. But it only came out of this caring heart. There didn't have to be words. It seemed to be that if one person made this heart connection with another, and really cared, there was a benefit that could come from that.

That's the kind of thing that undergirds my saying "stuff happens." And there's nothing particularly mystical about that. Whatever this means in terms of what we call the Divine Mystery, it raises a whole set of other questions. Because we have these simplistic, anthropomorphic ideas of what this Divine Mystery is, it sometimes blocks our ability to see what's really going on. We limit what's possible on the basis of our belief system.

PD: What's the conclusion you draw from that? If, as an intelligent, rational person, you say "stuff happens," and we get away from this mechanistic view of the world, what do we end up with then in terms of the potential for healing?

WI: I think one thing is that anyone can be a healer, that anyone has that capability if they are able to love another person. Like a child coming and loving a mother and laying a hand on her, that's as much a healing possibility as anything that might be done liturgically. It's that kind of thing that goes on in the human scene that is the potential for caring for one another, and it's a rationale for community. A community that cares for each member and that looks out for the best interest of each member, that's where balance – which is what health is, not the absence of all the negativity but rather a balance – can best happen.

PD: Flora, you were very careful not to say cure when you talked about wholeness and of healing a condition.

FL: Yes. We, in the Christian church, believe that healing is really the restoration of a relationship with God. And sometimes that involves physical cure and sometimes it may not. I mean, the ultimate healing may be in the dying. But if we're really speaking here about helping the living, and trying to restore the balance of spirit, soul, and body, we have to acknowledge that, as human beings, we are not separated parts. Our spirit being, our mental, our emotional, and our physical being are all interwoven and interconnected. And so something that interferes with our well-being at one level affects us at other levels. We experience this in our ordinary daily life.

PD: Sure, and that puts us out of balance.

FL: Yes. And we know that the intention of the universe, God's intention for us, is health and wholeness and balance, and that we are all interconnected in this cosmic web that we speak of today. And so we can be agents of healing or of "dis-ease," creating "dis-ease" for another, by the quality of our energy that interacts in this great cosmic web: between ourselves and the planet, between ourselves and creatures, and between each human.

PD: Were you skeptical at first? Have you seen cases that have just overwhelmed you?

FL: You mean crutches being thrown away and that kind of thing?

PD: No, not so much that, but just where people recover a balance.

FL: Oh yes. And I have seen healing in death.

PD: That's interesting to think of healing coming through death. Can you explain that?

FL: Well, a very personal incident. My 28-year-old son, who had never been sick a day in his life, was diagnosed with non-Hodgkin's lymphoma. And in spite of all traditional and non-traditional interventions and much prayer, Bryan was overcome by the disease 18 months later.

But in those intervening months, there was much healing that took place within his spirit, his mind, and his emotions. He had been ravaged by the attack of the disease and the most aggressive chemotherapy that could be given him, so therefore a great deal of his body's ability to fight back and overcome the disease was destroyed through that. But he died, I believe, with more peace than he had known in his living:

peace in relationships, peace with the sense of his belonging to the universe and to a Divine Love that is bigger than the short span of years we spend in this dimension.

So I know from that intimate experience with my son, painful as that was and is, the love carriers that we can be, the love and light bearers that we can be. For us, in the Christian church, there's a connection with the Divine light. Jesus said, "I am the light of the world." Jesus is the light bearer that we follow.

PD: Wayne, how skeptical were you when you started out on this?

WI: I think I would say that I was skeptical of the things that I saw in other traditions and on television. I did not really know what was going on, for example, when people would swoon. And yet I had observed that sort of thing happen once in a while, even in some instances when I was praying for a person. I interpreted it in non-mystical terms, believing that there was some psychological balancing going on. But I came to understand that they were surrendering themselves into something else, letting go. It was a spiritual thing. And I came to recognize that there was some important healing work going on in them.

There have been moments in my own experience when I have certainly felt ecstatic things, or felt elation beyond words, and I recognize that these are all part of a continuum. They're part of the spectrum of human experience, and sometimes we can help people get in touch with this breadth of spiritual possibility.

PD: And that then leads to...?

WI: Sometimes that can lead to a change of direction in life, when people recognize that reality is broader than they thought before, that it's grander than they thought it was. Therefore, they have to rethink their whole outlook.

FL: And I think, too, it's a big step, at least it was for me, to realize that the God of my childhood – the remote judge somewhere – was not a true concept. The truth is that God is within and among. And the nature of God, I'd heard all my life, is love. A big step for me was to become a meditator, to sit still long enough, to stop the busyness in my head, and to become quiet enough to sense the presence. Many people today are finding out the benefits of meditative practice, whether they come at it from a secular or religious point of view – both can be spiritual, depending on the intent.

We have a religious language around it and there is a difference. We believe, as Christians, that we don't go into a great void. We go into a loving presence whose name we call God, or the Christ presence. But we all experience benefits of that at every level of our being. I began to realize that meditating brought me to a center of myself. That helped me understand that I am essentially a spiritual being. And in the loss of my son Bryan, and parents, and brother, and others, I've become aware that, as essentially spiritual beings on a human journey, we're all spirits walking. And so in healing prayer, what we're really doing is connecting with the Divine essence in the other. The healing is already there. We're like a catalyst that helps get through the blocks so that that healing can manifest itself fully in the other.

So to me, there were some paradigm shifts that affected both my faith and my understanding of spirit connection.

PD: I think it was Schweitzer who said we all have a doctor within us. There's a Buddhist flavor to finding God "within."

FL: The Bible says we are, each one, a temple of the Holy Spirit. Each great religion has come to its connection with the Divine.

WI: Joseph Campbell's comment about this kind of thing has appealed to me. He says that whoever goes deeply into their own tradition will encounter whoever else has gone deeply into theirs. So whether we're Buddhist or whatever, when we go there we meet each other because we are in touch with the same spirit. It's not a different spirit, it's the same essence. We name it from our particular tradition, we approach this elemental mystery with the particular metaphors that are appropriate for our culture and tradition, but it is what's underneath it that is important. It's all pointing to what we in the United Church call "the Christ."

The analogy I like, as Campbell says, is that our tendency is to do as the person does who goes into the restaurant and opens the menu. It says filet mignon, and so the person tears that out and eats it without realizing that it's referring to something in the kitchen. Well, that's what happens sometimes with folks and religion. They go in and think, "This story is it." But that story is attempting to describe something beyond describing, and which is also being lifted up with other stories in other traditions.

PD: I've been reading about a level of Buddhist meditation where, as you inhale, you think of the suffering of someone, and, as you exhale, you send feelings of wholeness and health and security to that person. That's not unlike the idea of

Christ taking upon himself the sins of the world.

WI: Yes, and that method certainly fits with our understanding of what we're doing when we make a heart connection with someone.

PD: Is there a scientific explanation for what you call that "heart connection"?

WI: A couple of things come to mind. One is the book, from 1972, on the secret life of plants. The chap who invented the lie detector put his sensors on a rhododendron that was in his room and observed that when he had an emotional response to something, the machine went off and that his rhododendron was reading him. And that book describes a whole variety of experiments. There are things like that which are fascinating.

Gregory Bateson is the one who said that science doesn't prove anything, and yet we get all hung-up on the idea that it proves everything. He says the problem is that every scientific theory is based on an assumption that can't be proven, and therefore science cannot prove anything. It can only probe and suggest that statistically this looks like it's true. I think that's worthwhile remembering in terms of science. It's not our "god" either. It's useful, but there are those who use science to dismiss things and to say if it isn't scientific it's not feasible or possible or usable. And that's not good enough either. It's just a cop-out.

PD: We live in an age when science has been elevated, though, to being almost the only deliverer of truth, don't we?

WI: Well, we're coming past it.

PD: Do you think so?

FL: Now we have scientists who are exploring prayer with experiments, and doctors who are praying for their patients, and theologians who are laying on hands for healing. So a wonderful integration between the disciplines is beginning to happen today.

WI: There was the great separation back at the time of Descartes when they essentially said, "From now on we'll think of mind and body as separate, even though we can't prove it." So that allowed science to separate from the church and to get on with its narrow idea of what was okay.

Now we're recognizing that mind and body are not disconnected. They're part of the same entity – one on one end, one on the other. Like the north and south poles on a magnet; there's nowhere that you can say here's where south stops and here's where north begins. It's the same way with mind and body. We're in an exciting period, but it's pretty threatening. It can be threatening for the institutions and the establishment. The church is threatened by this, the medical people who have a mechanistic view are threatened by this.

I mean, what if we were able to cure people with prayer? I took my mother into McMaster Hospital to have some surgery and I was sitting around looking at this massive building predicated on people being ill and needing surgery. I thought, now, if we all came in here and prayed for everybody and they all got better and walked home, look at all the people who'd be out of work. This wouldn't be okay in our society.

PD: Do you think with the right power of prayer, that would be possible?

WI: No!

PD: Okay. Just checking!

WI: I don't think that, in the grand scheme of things, that's probably what it's all about. I think the illnesses and ailments and difficulties and struggles that we go through are all part of our learning, and that there exists a rationale for that kind of experience. Nirvana is not the absence of the negative. It's the balance between the two. I believe that suffering is somehow one of the ingredients of joy, that without the profound experience of suffering, you don't have a sense of what ecstasy is all about.

PD: Would it be fair to say that healing through prayer can be physical, but it is more likely to be emotional or mental?

WI: Well it certainly can be physical.

FL: Certainly!

WI: I think that there are earthquake experiences where some people are just poised for healing. They come to the church and they come forward and someone prays for them and they are suddenly changed. One person I remember had never had anybody ever pray for her before and she just melted in the compassion of that.

FL: There is a moment of receptivity when sometimes there is a profound breakthrough. Also, there are people who have experienced healings who have no faith themselves and who have been absolutely startled. We cannot ever tie it down. We're dealing here with the Divine Mystery, and so our task is to pray and the outcome we leave with God. We pray as best we know: we may use words, we may use pictures, we may use no words. But we use loving intention to help and to heal, according to what is moving that person toward health and wholeness, however that looks. We don't pre-scribe how that should look.

PD: Do you pray for a general well-being, or can it be more specific?

WI: It can be more specific, but our tendency is to pray for what we call God's highest good. There was some interest-ing work done by a group called Spindrift, in Pennsylvania, where they were doing prayer experiments with seedlings and such things, because the outcome could be seen rather quickly and also because this was a way of avoiding the pos-sibility that suggestion was involved. This was a double blind experiment in which there were other seedlings not receiv-ing prayer. The researchers found that among the plants that were prayed for, there was a significant difference in the outcome. It depended on how the researchers prayed.

I am referring to prayer that is specific and prayer that is not specific. They observed that if they prayed and asked for a specific kind of thing to happen for these plants, there was a benefit, but it wasn't as great as when they asked for God's highest good.

I think that's part of our human experience, too. We tend to dictate what the answer should look like and when we don't see that answer, we say there's been no answer. In reality, it's such a complex thing that the benefit may well be something emotional or mental or something else that doesn't manifest itself in the way we were expecting.

FL: Very often God works through process rather than through the spectacular breakthrough of the moment.

WI: But I think that's reasonable because that's how we grow. The spectacular stuff can be pretty scary. The gentle approach is what is long-lasting.

FL: Prayer with loving intentionality brings a healing response. It relieves pain and it enables a sense of well-being thereby releasing that healing mechanism that is innate within us.

PD: I'm struck by the similarities between music therapy and what you're saying about compassion. It's as if, like music, compassion allows us to be who we are again. Does that make sense?

FL: Perfect sense. Just like every color is a certain vibration, every emotion is a certain vibration, and we know about the wonderful healing vibration of love.

What does everybody need? We need to know that we're cared for, that we're worthwhile, that we're unique individuals, and that we're not alone in this world or left alone in the universe. We have a Divine connection.

PD: You know, that keeps coming up, that people feel increasingly isolated and alone.

WI: Yes, and I think there's technology in all of that. People are in front of their computer screens and are in relationship electronically with others, but they're isolated in other ways. Our culture is bringing that about, so there is certainly a role for the church and for communal gatherings where people come together because they have some common interest. There's a reason for those organisms to exist.

That, to me, is a beginning of the manifestation of John's vision in the book of Revelation in the Bible, where he describes the day when the city will exist but there will be no temple in it. John's vision is a picture of the better outcome, when the way we're to be is written inside of us and we're living it out without there having to be these traditional structures. The more we can live into that, the more we can get free of all that separates us and isolates us and gives us ammunition for being judgmental of each other.

We have a responsibility to work with people and to do what we can without it being a comment that we, or our methods, are any better than others.

FL: This is where we are and what we feel called to be about in our little corner of the world. But we know that there are other things happening in other places which are also effective for people. In my own journey, I've been around a little bit looking for nurture and the experience of the Divine. And now it's wonderfully exciting to me that there is this movement within the church, this openness, and this renewed sense of the gracefulness that is in our Christian story. And it's wonderful to see the healing and the joy that can happen there.

Chapter 5

BODY LANGUAGE

The Healing Touch of *Rochelle Graham*

❧

❧

Three years ago, Rochelle Graham offered her first workshop on British Columbia's Sunshine Coast. Since then, she has trained well over 100 people in the art of Healing Touch. A year ago, a group in Kelowna asked Rochelle to come and give a four-hour session. Nobody thought it would be necessary to limit attendance. Perhaps there were second thoughts when 75 people showed up! Recently, she returned to the same group in Kelowna and discovered that they now have three or four sessions a week during which they practice Healing Touch on each other!

After speaking with Rochelle, I'm sure she's a wonderfully gifted teacher and healer, but I'm just as sure she'd be the first to agree that the tremendous response by people to the practice of Healing Touch goes beyond her abilities alone and is really about our profound and increasing search for inner wellness.

I think, to some degree, it is also about reclaiming our bodies and our own health, about putting ourselves back in the driver's seat on the long road to healing.

Whether it's a baby's body that rejects a transplanted organ or seven bodies exploding in a spacecraft over the coast of Florida, we are all reminded, occasionally, that technology has its limits.

What I find compelling about the work of healers such as Rochelle Graham is the recognition of the mysterious power that already exists within each of us. Part of that mystery and excitement is not yet knowing the limits of our own ability to heal ourselves and others.

❧

PD: Do you do a lot of workshops now?

RG: Every weekend!

PD: Really?

RG: Three weekends a month I'm away teaching, and sometimes during the week.

PD: What kind of people attend your workshops? What do you see when you look out at the audience?

RG: Among professionals, it ranges from health care workers to social workers to bankers – all professions really. And then there are lots of lay people. People who are hungry for something else.

PD: Hungry for something other than, what? Traditional medicine?

RG: I think so. I think they feel as if they've come to the edge of their understanding of what health is, it's not satisfying them. And I mean health in a holistic sense, not just physical health.

I would say they are also spiritually seeking. A lot of the workshops I teach are in churches. I teach courses

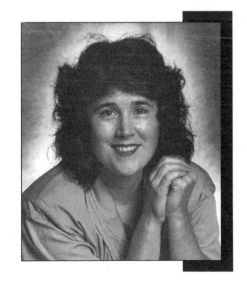

within congregations and people are flocking to them.

PD: Obviously there's a real demand for this kind of knowledge.

RG: Well, for example, I was in Red Deer not that long ago, at a United Church congregation, and 51 people signed up for the workshop, with ten on the waiting list.

PD: What do you teach them at these workshops?

RG: I teach them that there is more to us than the physical. There's an energy field around us, and whether it's named in Christian terms, biblical terms, or scientific terms, there is a force that moves through us, that nourishes us, and that is more than us. And then I teach them Healing Touch techniques, and that's what the rest of the weekend is, learning techniques from various healers.

PD: Can you actually see that aura around people, that energy field?

RG: I can see that. I can't see it all the time, but usually, if I'm teaching a workshop or working on someone, I see it.

PD: So it's clear colors and it gives you information?

RG: Definitely.

PD: Was that frightening, the first time you recognized that energy field?

RG: I would say so. One of the things you become aware of, as you begin to journey on this path, is that you're stretched continually. So you're always asking, "What is this?" And there's new learning that is frightening. The skeptic in me is always very present and is always asking what this is about.

PD: So it's always a bit uncomfortable, is it?

RG: Yes, I would say so.

PD: How did you get started?

RG: I was raised with parents who were traditional Anglicans but who also had more of a mystical philosophy about life. I was raised with a belief in hands-on healing and auras.

I worked as a physiotherapist at the Charles Camsell Hospital, in Edmonton, which at that time was the federal government native hospital. One of the fellows I worked with had ankylosing spondylitis, rheumatoid arthritis and rheumatic fever, all clinically diagnosed and I couldn't do much as a physio. I was not helping him and, in fact, he was getting worse. He signed himself out of the hospital, I thought, to die.

He came back a month later and he was fine. We had developed enough of a rapport that he shared with me that he had gone to see a medicine man. Through this patient, I was able to meet that medicine man. Over the course of five years during the 1970s, I spent time with this medicine man. But I just could not fit it into my world. I mean, that was really when it was frightening.

PD: What were you learning, what did you see that didn't fit into your world?

RG: Certainly the hands-on healing was not something that was acceptable from the medical perspective that I worked in. The belief system, the whole cultural aspect of sweat lodges and some of the rituals felt very much like a *Dances with Wolves* type of life to me. And it was, split between two worlds.

The irony of it is, at that point, I was married to a man who was doing his residency in family practice at the Royal Alexandra Hospital in Edmonton, and now that elder is on staff at that hospital.

PD: The elder you spent time with?

RG: Yes, he's now elder-in-residence at the Royal Alex.

PD: That's quite a growth isn't it? And a recognition, more than anything, I guess?

RG: Oh, it is! And that elder has also been given the Order of Canada for his work. For me, personally, it's wonderful to see that.

PD: How did it finally make sense and fit into the professional life that you had built for yourself?

RG: Well, I was working on the palliative care unit at St. Paul's Hospital, in Vancouver, and met a nurse who had just come from Toronto and who taught Therapeutic Touch. So I took a course from her. That was when, finally, I put the pieces together. Finally I had found a way that I could express it within my professional life.

PD: I would think that your idea of what healing means

has gone through as great a transformation as have your abilities as a healer.

RG: And still transforming!

PD: It seems to me that what we understand as health in North America has been so narrow. We're either healthy or unhealthy. We don't leave much room for subtleties. What does it mean to be healed, for you, now?

RG: Let me give you an example. Over the period of a year, I saw a few times a woman who was diagnosed with breast cancer and who had had surgery. I had first met her when she took one of my classes. Throughout that year, she began to explore old wounds – emotional wounds, spiritual wounds, relationship wounds – and she began to bring closure to those. She began to heal, coming to a place of resignation or resolution or acceptance.

Several months before she died, I was giving her a ride from Kelowna to Vancouver. She knew that the cancer had spread throughout her body but she looked at me and said, "I have never been healthier."

PD: What a moment.

RG: I just took it in, and for me, she was whole. She had come to that place of wholeness. She was absolutely beautiful and radiant and was in such a healthy place.

PD: One of the things that I've read about Therapeutic Touch is that the success of it depends, in some measure, upon the development of the person as a healer. I wonder where you think you are now in that development, on that journey as a healer?

RG: I think I'm always feeling like a beginner, aware of how much I've grown. But it feels like the more I'm aware of that, the more I'm also aware of how far there is to go.

And I believe, as a society, we're just beginning to explore how abundantly we can live. One of the workshops that I teach with two other people at Naramata Centre is called "New Life and Abundant Care." The principle behind it is that the more we begin to heal ourselves, the more abundantly we can live, and therefore the more we can be present for somebody else. And I know that I'm only beginning to explore the possibilities of how much life we can live.

PD: I heard someone, just last night, say we are moving into "the age of the heart."

RG: Yes, definitely. And that's fundamental for me in terms of the healing that I teach.

PD: In what way is that fundamental, how does that manifest itself in your teaching?

RG: Well, one of the things that I have studied is all the different cultures and their reference to heart, whether it be in native spirituality, in the Bible, or in Baha'i. All the cultures and religions that I have studied speak about the importance of the heart. So I began an exploration of the meaning of heart.

According to The Interpreter's Dictionary of the Bible, it's the connection to God, whatever that means for people.

But I believe it's through the heart that we connect to that power source.

PD: And to each other?

RG: And to each other. When we have moved to that place, we connect.

One of the examples I like to use is the difference between plugging into a socket in the wall and going to the source of power at the dam. We connect at a much deeper level, to a whole other level of energy, wisdom, and light. And when we do it from our hearts, it's not coming from us, but really through us.

PD: You've mentioned your faith a lot and I wonder how it is woven into the fabric of the healer you've become. It sounds like it's a fundamental element of your healing work.

RG: It is. It's fundamental, and it's getting stronger. I don't think it has a particular form, but as I connect more and more into my heart center and begin to connect with other people's hearts, I guess I'm connecting more with whatever that source is. And it expresses itself more through me, if that makes sense.

PD: It makes you more powerful as a healer, you mean?

RG: Yes, definitely.

PD: So is healing a sacred act for you?

RG: Yes, it is a sacred act, but I have evolved into that.

PD: It didn't feel like that at first?

RG: Not to the extent it does now. At first, I wouldn't have used the term "sacred."

PD: Aside from the actual technique of Therapeutic Touch, I understand that the intention of the healer is critical. When you sit down to do this with someone, what is your intention?

RG: My intention is to be an instrument. When I address myself to that source of healing energy, what I say is, "Let me be an instrument of healing." I imagine that I am an open vessel, allowing that to flow through me to the other person.

PD: "That" being what, specifically?

RG: I like to refer to it as energy and light. But energy, I guess, while acknowledging that there are different spectrums to that energy.

PD: How do you know that it works?

RG: By the results! By the healing and the life changes that I see happen. One of the things that I read – I guess it was an Alcoholics Anonymous book that I picked up – talked about various people's spiritual experience and how we can't judge that. All that matters is the fruit of that labor. So what matters for me is how that person has changed. In whatever happened between us, how is that person different?

PD: Are there people who really stand out for you as evidence of the power and influence you can have as a healer?

RG: One in particular is a woman who had severe fibromyalgia who, when I first started seeing her, could barely get up in the morning. Her mother had to help her. She began to recover fairly quickly. About six months later, in October, her son took his life while on drugs. Anyway, she saw me quite frequently right after that, and saw her physician in February. And her physician asked her, "What have you been doing? In the time that I would normally be putting people on medication, you've come off five medications."

Both she and her mother believe the only reason she is alive is because of Healing Touch. For myself, I just see the way this woman is now out in the world and doing things. Not that she hasn't grieved her son and isn't grieving her son, but she is now able to be productive and healthy and out helping other people. So whatever went on, there was a transformation that took place.

PD: Is there a connection between her openness to healing and the death of her son, do you think?

RG: Say more about that.

PD: Well, I'm wondering about the effect that the death of a loved one has on a person. I think Paul Simon says, in one of his songs, that the wind blows through his heart. I think death opens your heart up to the world in a way that makes it as vulnerable as it's likely ever to be. And I wonder if that doesn't then welcome in the powers of healing.

RG: I think so. She had already begun that process or she wouldn't have come. But I have no doubt about what you say. Another friend of mine just suffered quite a severe heart attack and had to have open heart surgery, and the transformation in that woman from that broken heart is amazing.

PD: It's almost as if our bodies have to get our attention, isn't it?

RG: I believe that. I believe our body is our greatest teacher and it will teach.

PD: It's strange that we've become so removed from the language of our body.

RG: I think that we, as a culture, have moved into our heads, into our intellect to such an extent, that we have disconnected ourselves from our bodies. I'm not a theologian, but my understanding of what has often happened in religion is that it has very much cut us off from our bodies. Too often, we have sought the source of God outside of us rather than inside of us.

PD: At some price. We've paid a price for that separation.

RG: Yes.

PD: So is healing, in a sense, recovering that connection for you?

RG: That's a major focus of what I teach people – not just when I'm teaching in a class, but also when I'm working one-to-one with someone. What is your body feeling? What is it telling you? Can you feel my hands here? Are they feeling warm? Can you feel that warmth begin to move through your body?

And for some people that's a difficult task.

PD: Because they're not open to it?

RG: No, I could give you examples of different types of illnesses. Certainly the cases of fibromyalgia and chronic fatigue that I've worked with, their legs feel like concrete to me.

PD: Really?

RG: So for them to begin to move energy or warmth through their bodies when they haven't felt warmth in their legs for so long...

PD: So is that a lost cause for you?

RG: Oh no, I've worked quite successfully with those illnesses.

PD: I guess I better ask you how you do it, when someone comes to see you?

RG: Well, if it's the first time someone comes to see me, I do what I call an intake history. Then I get their medical background. What I'm specifically looking for is what damage has happened to their energy field.

PD: From physical injury?

RG: It could be physical injury, it could be surgery that they've had, it could be an emotional wound. What I want to know is whether there is an area of the body that has received perhaps more insult than other places.

PD: And once you have that information?

RG: Then I put them on my table – which is like a massage table – and I do what I call an energetic assessment, feeling all the layers of the energy. What I'm perceiving through my hands, through my eyes, and sometimes just through my gut reactions and intuitive senses, helps me form a picture of what's going on.

PD: Is it stressful for you when you come upon wounds?

RG: No, it's not stressful. It would have been if I hadn't done so much of my own healing. I just feel fully present for that person and their offering.

PD: I guess we all carry around our wounds, but I wonder if you're finding the results of physical or emotional trouble, or can it be something that is still to come, that hasn't manifested itself yet?

RG: It can be something still to come that hasn't manifested itself physically, although usually the body shows it in some way. It may not be to the extent that it has stopped them.

PD: Right. What do you do when you find an area like that?

RG: I make a choice on what kind of treatment I need to do. Is it a full-body treatment or is it going to be just a localized area that needs to be worked on? For most of the people I see, it's full-body treatment and we're engaging in some kind of long-term work.

That's when I would use some of the techniques of other healers – *chakra* connection or Barbara Brennan's full-body chelation. And, for a lot of people, they are hungry for a healthy touch. So certainly something like *chakra* connection is a really good one to start with.

Through all our joints and as well as the seven energy centers on the body – the *chakras* – we can receive energy. So it's simply a matter of placing your hands on those centers, moving from the feet up to the heart, and then from the arms into the heart. It's a fundamental technique in the Healing Touch program.

PD: Are there situations where you understand there is nothing you can do?

RG: Yes, definitely. An example would be a man that I worked on who was a draft dodger and who had so much anger towards the U.S. government, that it was filling his field and, I believe, was a big source of his chronic pain. And so I asked him if he was able to let go of that anger and he said, no, that it was the only thing keeping him alive.

PD: The energy of that anger?

RG: Right.

PD: So he was conscious of that?

RG: He was aware of that.

Another situation involved someone who came to me with whiplash following a car accident. The settlement and court case was two years away. I asked him, "Are you able to heal before the court case?" And he said "no."

PD: I guess that's the openness of the client?

RG: That's right. I mean, I probably could have kept seeing him, but I didn't feel it was worth either my time or his and that he probably would be better off seeing a physiotherapist who would do regular physio. He wasn't really ready to investigate some of the deeper issues around his neck.

PD: That's one of the things I've been thinking about. That is, if I'm not well, in whatever way, I have to understand that true healing is only going to be mine if I become intimately involved in the process.

RG: Exactly.

PD: And I realize now that the kind of health that comes from surgery, or from a bottle of pills, may be necessary in the immediate sense, but it's only a stopgap.

RG: And we see that all the time in the hospitals when people get readmitted. The initial problem may be solved, but another one surfaces very quickly.

PD: Where do you think Healing Touch and Therapeutic Touch belong in the larger medical picture?

RG: I like to call them complementary. They aid in relaxation, they aid in pain relief, and they provide a level of comfort and caring.

Our belief at St. Paul's Hospital is that anybody who's in contact with the patient can do this, so now, even the lab techs are doing some "unruffling," or clearing of the energy field, before they poke a person. A pastoral care worker or a social worker and I might work together, one on either side of the patient, doing *chakra* connection. What we find is that the person will open up and begin to talk a lot more about what is happening for them, and be able, then, to receive something. When we first did this, the social workers were amazed at what the clients would begin to reveal.

PD: You know, it sort of struck me as you were talking just then that the human mind, when it thinks someone else actually cares for us, can be really powerful.

RG: Oh it is. One of the things we do when we do this work is to be fully present for another human being. And that is rare.

In this workshop I just taught, "New Life and Abundant Care," we asked, "How do we feel when someone is fully present for us?" The feelings that came out were, "I feel respected, I feel worthy, I feel loved that someone's caring enough to spend that amount of time with me." So that's definitely a part of it.

There's a belief within me – I don't know if it's a belief or an experience – that when we begin to access the realms of energy and healing through the heart, it will take our heads a while to catch up. It just becomes frustrating for me if I get too much into my head trying to figure it out. I stay more in the experience.

There's an interesting phrase that I use when I teach within the churches. It's from Ephesians and it speaks about when you bring Christ into your heart through faith, and you allow that power to flow through you, it will be beyond knowledge.

It's my life work. This is no longer a job for me and I don't mean that lightly. What's fascinating for me is that I've been in and out of churches all my life, but I never would have considered myself someone who would have called this a ministry. And yet, that's what I now call this; this is a ministry of healing for me. I have said I will go wherever I'm called, and that's what I do.

PD: Do you ever think, "Boy, look at how far I've come, where might this lead me?"

RG: Oh yes! And I get scared! I mean, that's the edge that I live on. Where is this going and what am I being called to do? But also, the absolutely exciting possibilities. My life now is seeing those possibilities, seeing the transformation that occurs in a community of people.

One of the typical things about congregations is that people aren't open to each other. They have masks on, it's not a place where you can be broken. And what I see happening is that transformation – people moving into brokenness, the spontaneous hugging that begins to happen, their hearts opening to each other. That in itself is quite miraculous! We can't begin to imagine the impact that will have on our health, on our wholeness, and on our relationships.

Chapter 6
A STILL LIFE

The Contemplative Healing of *Father Tom Ryan*

☙

This conversation with Father Tom Ryan reminded me of a kind of parable the Pulitzer Prize-winning Harvard psychiatrist John Mack told me one night in Boston. It seems a church came into millions of tax-free dollars but was unsure of what to do with the glorious windfall. In search of expert advice, the church committee looked up the phone number of economist Milton Friedman. When asked how the church should deal with the millions, Mr. Friedman quite quickly advised that they should give it all away to the most needy among us. Stunned, the church official stammered, "Is this the real Milton Friedman?"

"Is this the real church?" came the reply.

I thought of that again because there is, to me, something very "real" and compelling about Tom Ryan and the indomitable spirit and energy of his faith. I first met him, for a television program, a few years ago, and I liked him a lot almost immediately.

Tom Ryan seems wisely understanding of the tendency in North America to fill so much of our lives with stuff that really doesn't matter – ambition, greed, consumerism, and so on. I find his sensitivity, to spiritual homelessness for example, rare, and it explains why he is no stranger to healing, having spent 14 years as Director of the Canadian Centre for Ecumenism. He is now Director of an ecumenical center for spirituality and Christian meditation called Unitas, located in the stunning former McConnell family home and Benedictine monastery nestled serenely on the side of Mount Royal in Montreal.

It's still a bit curious to me, but I think the profound silence within those exquisite tapestry-draped walls can be as healing as any conversation that takes place there.

PD: Let's start with your journey to this home and your belief in ecumenism. You said, when you were on your sabbatical studying in the East, that something streaked with a psychic effect across your consciousness. Can you explain that?

TR: The context for that experience was a sabbatical in 1991 in India, following the World Council of Church's General Assembly in Canberra, Australia. As I went and lived in ashrams and Buddhist monasteries and so forth, I kept running into people from the West – particularly people in their 20s, 30s, and 40s. The conversation would inevitably turn to, "Well, what brought you here? What are you doing here?" And inevitably the response came back along these lines: "Christianity doesn't teach practical methods, means, or supports for my spiritual journey, my spiritual growth and development, so I've come here. I'm looking for a teacher and they're teaching me yoga, they're teaching me how to meditate, they're teaching me how to breathe, they're teaching me how to fast and how to do all this in the context of my God quest."

And as I listened, I felt profoundly challenged by that as a Christian and as one in a position of Christian teaching. And I think the end of my own discernment along those lines was a recognition that, yes, we perhaps do a much better job of talking about faith and love than actually helping to...

PD: Provide the tools?

TR: Yes. Provide the tools, teach people what it means, in concrete terms, to love and to be committed to prayer and to be a disciple and to really spell out some concrete, practical means and ways of expressing that.

And there were two moments in that whole unfolding of experience. One came in a Hindu ashram in Tiruvanumali. While I was meditating in that ashram in the temple of prayer, my mind was open and receptive and it came in really strong and clear: this sense of call, of mission, of being sent to go and found, or to open, or to help get up and going an ecumenical center for spirituality when I got back home.

It was to be a place where the pathways to God and all the religious traditions of the world could be set out on the table, and the covers taken off and competent instruction could be provided and people could come and be fed and be nourished.

And about a month later, I was in Dharmsala on a course in Buddhist meditation method and doctrine. Again, I was sitting still in meditation one day and it came like a shooting star across the screen of my consciousness and landed with a thud. It was so clear that I journaled about it after both experiences. Both times, I described the experience, and by the time I came back, I was even starting to dream of where this could be and who might be interested in helping me with this.

PD: It was that clear and detailed for you?

TR: Oh yes. And one of the first things I did when I got back home was to call one of the members of my own community – the Paulists – and say, "I really had this strong inspiration while I was there, and this is where it's running, and I thought of you as somebody who might resonate with that. I'd like to lay it out for you and see whether it strikes any chords of interest with you." And so we talked about it.

But what I had in mind was a location my own community owns an hour and a half outside New York City. It's in the woods, on a lake – a very sylvan, idyllic setting for that sort of thing.

Then I came back here to Montreal and I discovered that, in my absence, the Benedictines had left the house and turned the property and building over to the archdiocese of Montreal. The archdiocese was looking for a new vocation for the house in continuity with its former vocation as a place of prayer in the midst of the city, particularly where laity could enter into the contemplative dimension of Christian life.

Within a short time after my return, I was invited to sit on kind of a brainstorming committee to think about new possibilities: what could we do in this marvelous facility perched on the flank of the mountain just off the center of downtown Montreal, this little oasis?

So this group met and we shared ideas and so forth. It was between the first and second meeting that, early one morning (I meditate twice daily and have done so for 20 years), it just kind of bubbled up from my subconscious: was I supposed to make a connection between what happened in India and the availability of this house? Now it may seem strange that I hadn't made the connection to that point, but I just hadn't. I'd been thinking in other terms. I'd been thinking of woods and lakes and so forth, and, all of a sudden, the idea of perhaps using this house just bubbled up. "Is this from the Holy Spirit?" And I said, "Well, there's only one way for me to find that out and that is to put the idea out to the others and see how they respond."

PD: I wanted to ask a bit more about those – I don't know if "visions" is too strong a word – but about when this came to you in the East. I think you've written that it's one thing to receive those kinds of messages, it's quite another to know what to do with them.

TR: Exactly.

PD: So did you feel frightened or called as a healer at that point?

TR: I don't think healing was the context of my perception or my thought at that point in time, though I could reflect upon that now, in the light of what's happening here. I have a better sense, in the midst of it, of some of the very real healing processes that are at work.

I think the experience was one of recognizing that this has to happen because I was receiving so many things of value from my interface with Hinduism, Buddhism, and Islam. I was really feeling, at a very deep level, how much we have to share with one another as world religions and how much we need places where that kind of sharing can take place. So I think my reaction to it was more one of being stirred, of being excited by the prospect. But how does one begin? And where?

PD: Give me the sales pitch. How did you sell the idea for this house?

TR: Well, I just started off with the naked idea of making it an ecumenical center for spirituality which would, in a first phase, focus on throwing open the Christian treasure chest so that people could discover the broad range of traditions that are within Christianity. And then, once the Christian identity of the place had become clearly established, because I really think we need places that have a clear Christian identity in which to do this, and precisely because we are Christian, we would want to be open to whatever God is doing in other religions as well. I wanted all of that to be made available to people. Whatever is of wisdom and goodness and truth needs to be brought into our own purview and appreciation.

Basically, I just presented the idea of taking the tradition of Christian meditation that the Benedictines had rooted here and of building upon that, broadening it to include other ways of prayer, other pathways to God, of inviting people from the different Christian traditions to come and bring the gifts of their traditions with them, of setting those on the table, and of helping people appreciate and develop a taste for that more cosmopolitan cuisine.

So the way it happened was first at the level of the committee organizers. Then they suggested I talk with the Chancellor about this. I did and he was very taken with the ecumenical idea. He said, "I'd like you to put some of this in writing and spell it out a little more clearly." So I spelled out a kind of first, second, and third phase of development. Then he said, "I'd like you to take this and present it to those charged with the trusteeship of the building." So I did. And again, the response of all three was very positive. They were very encouraging and said, "We'd like you to talk with the Archbishop about this." Well, at that point, I started feeling severe tremors of trepidation within. I began to think, "Well, if he likes this idea, something could really happen here and am I prepared for it to happen?" You know what I mean? I had naively gone forward with the idea that I could present the vision, but that somebody else could come along and execute it.

So there I am, talking with the Archbishop of Montreal for a couple of hours one fine June day and he's saying things that are absolutely bowling me over. Here's somebody who grew up his whole life in a French Canadian context, with very minimal ecumenical exposure and experience. So for me to come in and propose that he share this plum spot with all the other churches in the city – I had no idea how he'd respond to this.

He listened intently and said, "You know, I have asked all the contemplative communities in the city to pray with us, that we might find a really fitting vocation for this house, and several proposals have been made, but they didn't move me. They didn't click and I just said, "No, not this, not this, not this." Then he said, "This is the first time I'm hearing something that really makes my heart leap up!"

PD: Do you know what it was that touched him in that way?

TR: Well, I think he is truly a person who understands and believes that God can work in many ways and he's very inclusive in his approach. I think he was excited by the idea. He had said, in his opening address, when he became Archbishop of Montreal, that he didn't just want to talk ecumenism, he wanted to do practical ecumenism. He wanted to find ways that the churches in this city could really act together. So I reminded him of that.

He was saying things like, "I would be the happiest man in the world if this vision could become concrete reality. I'll back you 150% on this." And all of a sudden I'm realizing he means exactly what he says! And he's saying, "I realize as I reflect on what happened under the Benedictines, that John Main was a very strong leader with a very clear vision and that leadership was key to how rapidly that grew, so would you be willing to give this five years of your life, to helping us get it up and going?" At which point I took a big, deep swallow and psychically, I think, began to do a rapid back pedal. "Now wait a minute! I'm not looking for a new job. I'm very happy in my job as Director of the Ecumenical Centre and they're not standing in line for that position! I'm not sure who would step in if I stepped out, blah, blah, blah."

And he said, "Okay. Well that's all right, I've heard enough for today. Let's just leave it there. The next step I'd like to take is to call all the other church leaders together and see how they respond to this idea." And that eventually happened during the week of prayer for Christian unity in 1993.

We had them all here for supper just to show them the house. And it was kind of funny. I'll never forget it because the tradition of entering into the meditation chapel is that everybody takes off their shoes like Moses before the burning bush. You're on holy ground. And so I discreetly suggested that they stay in custom with the tradition of the house in that respect, which they happily did. But then, I fully expected they would all go in and sit down in the choir stalls along the walls. Instead, they all headed for these Buddhist meditation cushions on the floor!

So here we've got the Cardinal Archbishop of Montreal, the Anglican Bishop, the United Church General Secretary, the Presbyterian Moderator, and the Armenian

Orthodox Primate of Canada all sitting cross-legged in their stocking feet on these Buddhist cushions!

PD: What have you done?

TR: And I said, "Here I am without a camera to capture this moment." It was one of those great icons, and there I was, in front of it!

PD: If it didn't originally feel like a "call" to heal, I sense now that you feel like this has become a home where healing can take place. How do you characterize that healing?

TR: Well, I think I always was aware, because of the ecumenical nature of Unitas, that this was a healing work on a very real level. I'm talking now about the healing of the churches. I've been working in ecumenism full-time the last 15 years and one of the things that has really struck me is the absence of places where Christians can actually come together and share faith and life, where they can come to an experiential appreciation of each other precisely as Christians, precisely as members of Christ's body.

At the same time, ecumenists everywhere are saying that the agenda for the next decade is sharing of faith and life at the grassroots level. But how is this to happen in any kind of ongoing way if people just remain in the enclaves of their own congregations and parish communities? So, early on, I was aware of how profoundly a work like this could contribute to the task of healing the wounds of division amongst the churches.

The dialogue commissions can only do so much in terms of resolving, on an intellectual level, the centuries-long church-dividing questions. But there's another whole level

that involves psyche and emotion and prejudice and his-
torical consciousness that can only be changed by people
meeting people and coming, through that encounter, to a
new perception of one another.

There is a vocation in our name Unitas. It obviously
speaks to the divided churches as a place where they can
come together and experience a deeper, more visible unity in
the body of Christ and mirror that to the world. But it is also
about more than just bringing Catholics and Protestants and
Anglicans and Orthodox and Evangelicals together.

Unitas is also about the unity of the various ethnic groups
in this city and in Canada. This is something that the French
and English in Montreal are working on together. All our
prayers and services are bilingual. Some of our programs are
offered in French, some in English, and at every level of our
organizational structure there's an easy flow back and forth
between the languages. That's part of the excitement of
Unitas, that it helps to provide a place where that kind of
healing can go forward as well.

Just last week, there was a group of French and English
meeting here for the purpose of building creative connections following the referendum experience, which was enor-
mously painful. There was some very frank sharing amongst
them as to their feelings of isolation and frustration, their
feelings of being disenfranchised. The group has decided to
continue meeting and I think Unitas is providing a very
special place for that. It means a great deal to them.

PD: I think you described it once as people feeling the "inner shove," as an action of the grace of God.

TR: That's right. I don't know whether you recall the Uncle

Remus story of Brer Rabbit and Tar Baby, in which Brer Fox, I think it was, creates a Tar Baby in the hopes of catching Brer Rabbit. Brer Rabbit comes along, sees the Tar Baby and says, "Hi!" When he doesn't get a response, he hits it. Of course his fist gets stuck in the tar. So he tries to pry it away and the other hand gets stuck in it. So he kicks it and his foot gets stuck in it. Finally, the other foot gets stuck in it. So there he is, totally stuck in it. I think that describes my present situation. I'm in! I'm in and it would be very hard to get out at this point.

PD: But you don't feel stuck do you?

TR: No, as a matter of fact, that's where the metaphor breaks down. It's definitely the most challenging, daunting, and difficult undertaking I've ever put my hand to, but, at the same time, it's glorious, it's energizing, and I feel an undercurrent of joy in it all.

I see three key notes in terms of the healing work taking place here. One would be ecumenical, which we've already mentioned – the healing of the churches as we act together, witness together, pray together, and live together in this place.

PD: That healing, though, doesn't mean agreement does it?

TR: No.

PD: The healing here invites diversity?

TR: And I think that's very consistent with the whole model of unity that the churches are pursuing. It's not a model of uniformity, it's not a model of the larger churches absorbing the smaller ones, or of churches of equal size coalescing. It's a model of unity in diversity, of looking for a common foundation on the essentials of the faith beyond which there can be freedom. Let there be diversity of expression and liturgical tradition and canonical organization, and let it all be perceived as so many jewels in the crown of the universal church which is truly catholic – small "c" – reflecting the richness of diverse cultures and traditions and mentalities.

There's a second kind of healing that takes place here and that has to do with the whole phenomenon of reconciliation of people who have been wounded by their own church and who are not ready yet to step foot inside a building with a steeple on it.

They are on a very real spiritual journey and have a real sense of God in their lives and are simply looking for a place and a group of fellow travelers with whom they can continue to explore. But they're not ready to do that in an explicitly ecclesial context.

We're providing a place where they can once again speak of Christ, where they can once again be a Christian and explore their own spiritual walk with others who may have had similar kinds of experiences, with people who may be in a rather ambiguous or marginalized position *vis-à-vis* their churches but who believe deeply, regardless.

Any number of people have said to me, "I've been looking for Unitas for years, even before it existed, and as soon as I stepped through the doors I had this experience of coming home." It's very powerful to hear people say that. So that's the second dimension.

PD: And the third?

TR: I'd say evangelization, which is also a very real work.

Let me tell one story to illustrate this.

In my first summer here, a little over a year ago now, this lovely blond girl walked in with a baseball cap on her head and a ponytail hanging out the back of her cap. She looked around and said, in hushed tones before meditation period, "Can I come in to meditate here?"

I said, "Sure." So she walked in and sat down on the cushion with that baseball cap on her head. She spent a quiet half hour that day and returned more and more regularly. And then she asked, "Can I come and spend a few days here?"

I said, "Sure, that's why we're here." So she came and spent a few days and it became three weeks. At supper, in our group around the table, the conversation would be about many things and one day a bishop was mentioned. She turned to me with all the naiveté of a child and asked, "What's a bishop?"

Now, here's a 35-year-old woman living in Quebec, Archbishop Turcotte had just been made a Cardinal, which was front-page news, and you wonder how could anybody living today not know what a bishop is?

This woman was baptized but was a perfect example of one in whom the seed was placed but in whom it had lain dormant all these years. And now, you can see how this seed is sprouting royally into something truly beautiful. She's become one of our chief friends of Unitas. She's helped us get government grants to pay workers to help with the house cleaning and the grounds keeping and even to get a cook in the kitchen. She is in the midst of a full blossoming of a natural contemplative vocation. This very week she's going off for a full week to a hermitage in the countryside somewhere. She is a very good example of what has happened for many people here.

People have simply come through the doors – drawn by a sense of the spiritual, understood in some vague way –

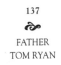
looking for something beyond the consumer lifestyle, beyond materialism, beyond the car and the house and what's on television tonight, looking for something more substantive, a still point at the center of their turning world.

So I've seen a lot of them come through our doors and it's like watching a plant grow under a grow light. You can literally see the difference from week to week. This woman I referred to is now reading Thomas Merton and *Seeds of Contemplation* and *Seven Story Mountain*. It's really exciting to see that.

PD: She came through the door, and I don't mean this in any critical way, but she came through the door with ignorance, not with prejudice.

TR: That's right.

PD: I'm also interested in the people who come through those doors with prejudice. To understand the healing that has to take place for those people, I guess it helps to understand the wounds which they feel.

TR: It's hard to generalize. For one person, it may have been a run-in with their pastor. For another, it may have been a position their church has taken with regard to women's ordination, or it may have been an experience they had in church one Sunday that left them with a sense that the people in church were hypocrites and that they didn't want to be among them. So people are wounded, alienated by different kinds of things. I think what we're trying to provide here is a safe, welcoming space where they can get out some of their anger, pursue healing, and explore questions of forgiveness and reconciliation. And at times, I find myself aware of the slow, steady suturing of the wounds in the body of Christ that is taking place here.

I was leading a group one day and, during the coffee break, I was standing and talking with three women. In the course of the conversation, I discovered that one was Antiochian Orthodox tradition, one was Anglican, and the third was United Church. And here I was, a Catholic priest. Even better, we'd all just shared this beautiful day of faith together. We were all profoundly aware of our solidarity with one another in this journey. We just sort of discovered, by-the-by, that we had come from four different pathways to this clearing in the forest. We just looked at each other and said, "Isn't this exciting! Here we are, we've just shared this day and we've all come from different churches and we're learning to see one another with new eyes!"

That, too, is a very real kind of healing. As people begin to see the world anew, there's a wholeness that's being restored to our vision as Christians. It's almost as if you take somebody with a cataract, whose sight is partially limited, and you give them laser therapy and they have an experience that enables them to see again with a new vision and appreciation for reality.

PD: I wanted to ask you a bit about the importance of prayer in your own life, because it seems to me that prayer or meditation is your scalpel in spiritual medicine. It's a very powerful tool for you, isn't it?

TR: I think the particular form of prayer that I introduce people to on the retreats and prayer days that I lead relates to the whole question of restoring balance. It's on that level where there's a real issue of healing.

I think, basically, people's lives today are off kilter and out of focus. We're sick with the speed of activism, of too many things to do. You and I have discussed these issues before, about why people work so much. The disciplines I invite people to consider for their lives are disciplines aimed at restoring balance in our living.

PD: A balance between?

TR: Well, I think any spirituality for our time, if it's to be authentic, has to be holistic. So if the dimensions of my life are emotional, spiritual, physical, psychological, and intellectual, then I want to look at each of those and ask: how's my balance here?

In terms of my intellectual life, am I reading good soul food with any kind of regularity, so as to keep turning over the soil of my mind to fresh inspirations and ideas? Am I being a good steward of the vessel given to me, in which I carry this treasure of the Divine life? Am I eating a balanced diet? Am I exercising regularly so as to really lead a vitalized existence, to have energy and enthusiasm and a positive response to life? Am I getting enough sleep? And so forth.

Then I look to the affective dimension of life. How much time do I take, on a regular basis, just to kick back and share life with friends? With people for whom I don't have to perform, with whom I can be who I am.

PD: And prayer opens the door to that kind of contemplation for you?

TR: The prayer we teach here is a meditative kind of prayer, it's a contemplative form of prayer and it comes from the earliest centuries of the Christian tradition. It basically invites the contemporary activistic citizen of the '90s, who probably spends most of his or her time conjugating the three verbs of doing, having, and wanting, to make some space in their life for a fourth: being. Being. Just entering into the joy of being – not doing "nothing," but learning to enter into creative non-doing.

PD: That's a very difficult lesson, isn't it?

TR: Very difficult.

That's one of the reasons why I teach yoga in conjunction with meditation. Yoga was, first of all, designed in order to prepare people to meditate better. But I also find that it speaks with particular appropriateness to the citizen of contemporary Western society, because it gives fidgety activists something to do while introducing them to an experience of inner quiet and stillness. You know, "Put yourself in this posture, enter into that stretching pose, and hold it! Be aware of what's going on in your body as you do it." So it's a very contemplative kind of exercise – it's meditation in motion – but it's also giving them something to do.

It's a kind of bridge experience. It makes it easier for people to enter into meditation. It's unrealistic to think that they can just come in off the streets and, all of a sudden, find the off switch and have a perfectly blank, blissful mind for the next 25 minutes. It doesn't happen that way. You've got to accept the fact that when you're going 100 miles per hour and you see a stop sign, you've got to start applying pressure to the brake lightly and bring yourself to a slow, steady, gradual stop, rather than all of a sudden throwing on the emergency brake and thinking it's going to suffice.

PD: I guess it's different for each person, but you must recognize now when healing is beginning. What are the signs of healing? When do you know something is being transformed?

TR: Well, let me tell you another story. One day a woman came in to see me about a difficulty. She was observing a pattern in her own behavior that she was very "dis-eased" about. She was a divorcee and she was lonely. She would go to bars after work in the evening, and occasionally, when she found somebody she liked, she would go home and spend the night with that person. She didn't respect herself for doing this. She wanted to break out of it, but she didn't know how.

I asked her if she knew how to meditate and whether she'd be interested in learning. She said, yes, she would. She didn't really understand how that was going to help, but if I thought it would, she'd be willing to take that on faith and to try. So I gave her some basic instruction in meditation and said, "If you're faithful to this, you'll begin to experience the change within you."

She came back about three months later and said, "You know, I have been meditating and I've found I can't go home with a guy and spend the night with him anymore. There's something within me now that demands a greater integrity, a greater honesty with myself, that demands that I act in a way that is more in harmony with the sacredness of what I'm discovering is within me."

I thought of her one day as I was sitting out in front of my little ashram hut in India. There was this "whoosh" and this big palm tree branch fell right at my feet. It was about 50 feet long. I looked up at the tree and I saw that new, green branches were coming out right at the top and gradually shading the ones beneath them. And as the ones beneath no longer received the sun, they turned brown and began to die and, under their own weight, began to fall.

There's a sense in which that's exactly what happened to her. By turning to a different kind of light on a regular daily basis, new branches started to grow up and to overshadow former patterns of behavior in her life. Eventually, because they were not getting light, energy, and attention anymore, they died and cracked off under their own weight.

I share that with you in the spirit of your question, "How does the change come?" It's subtle, but real. And generally, when people start to meditate, I say, "Commit yourself to this for ten weeks before you even evaluate whether this is worth doing or not."

PD: So it's process, isn't it?

TR: Yes.

PD: It's a new way of treating the spiritual system, I guess.

TR: That's right. I think it would be fair to say that there's a wound at the root of our being and we are constantly treating that wound. We're constantly administering salves and balms to it and trying to diminish the extent to which it handicaps us in terms of the kind of life we'd like to lead.

PD: Tell me about Taizé prayer.

TR: The Taizé prayer is a very contemplative form of prayer. It comes out of an ecumenical community in Taizé, France, which has become a Mecca for young people from around the world. On any day in the summer, you'll find a minimum of 5,000 young people from every continent in the world. It's a real happening in the Holy Spirit. It grew up under the aegis of five Brothers who simply started to live what they called "a parable of reconciliation." Again, that's a beautiful image for what we are trying to live here as well.

The aroma of what they were living went out, as it always will when something authentic starts to happen, and people caught the scent of it in the airways and followed their noses to it. And today, it's amazing to see the influence that Taizé has had, by virtue of the ripple effect, in the many places where Taizé prayer is practiced and entered into all around the world.

The prayer they've developed, I've come to recognize, really teaches people a way into contemplative prayer. It provides them with an experience of inner quiet and stillness.

Taizé prayer is essentially a very simple rhythm of short, one-line chants which are repeated for maybe three or four minutes. It becomes like a mantra and the function is the same. A mantra simply means a mental tool, an instrument by which you can control the flow of thoughts. It focuses the mind. It loads the consciousness with one thing so that, after you've sung it twice, the grasping, seeking, curious mind says, "All right, already! I've got the meaning. I know the meaning of this. Give me something else!" But you don't give it something else. You just keep repeating this song over and over. Eventually, the mind drops down beneath its general questing, curious level, to a deeper, intuitive level where it just rests in the meaning of the song.

Then the song drifts off and leaves you in silence for a few minutes. Then another song will come up, out of that silence, and you'll do the same thing again. You might repeat that for several chants. Then you'll just sit for a period of, maybe, ten minutes of quiet, in the course of which somebody will drop in, like a little drop of water into a still pond, a few verses of scripture. And you just take that in, in that rich tradition that the church calls *lexio divina*, just masticating the word in silence. And out of that, again, will come another chant. And that's really all it is!

It's very powerful and people are taken very deep in the prayer by virtue of the dynamic of the chanting and the silence and the ambience. There are a lot of little vigil candles all over the place and at one point a Taizé cross is placed on the floor. People are invited to come up and place their forehead on the cross as a way of symbolically giving their own concerns, hopes, fears, anxieties for the world and for others they love, and so forth to the crucified but risen Lord. It's very powerful to witness.

PD: Do you understand how it is that North Americans have become so frightened of silence? Surely that must act as an obstacle to healing.

TR: Definitely. I think there are some very deep forms of healing that can only come as a person learns to be still. And that ability to be still relates, as well, to their ability to be comfortable with who and what they are, to become who they are in a more conscious kind of way.

Certainly, a lot of the noise in people's lives today is a form of escape. It's a way for them to avoid facing what's inside them. To go away for a day, or a few days, or even to regularly take a half hour a day just to be still and know that God is God, or to come before the One Who Is in full, loving attention, or to just be alone with your own thoughts and to look at your own life – which is the essence of a retreat experience – is to have a willingness to come face-to-face with what is there. And to deal with it.

The dealing with it is the healing. It will come up if one simply provides the tranquil space and the environment. There will be healing. People regularly find that, if they just take the time to be still and to be quiet and to be reflective about what is going on in their lives, they will discover, in fairly short order, the answers to the questions they have about the next step, or what they need to do in order to get out of this feeling of disease or paralysis or whatever it might be.

Part of what happened, through the Protestant Reformation, was that all the monasteries were closed. The monasteries were the centers of silence, the contemplative retreat centers, and they were closed in all the regions where the reform went out. Abuses had crept in that needed correcting, but the baby was thrown out with the bath water. The Protestant traditions today are in the process of rediscovering that whole contemplative tradition and finding a very rich vein in it.

I think even in the Catholic tradition in the West, the contemplative tradition was lost to lay people in general, and even to the professionally religious, in what came to be judged as the heresy of quietism. That really meant that the contemplative tradition, particularly during the times of the Spanish Inquisition and the counter reformation, became suspect to the point where even the great mystics in the West – such as Ignatius of Loyola, John of the Cross, and Theresa of Avila – had to really watch their flanks. There were things they couldn't really say straight out for fear of being called on the carpet. As a matter of fact, Ignatius and John of the Cross spent time in prison and had to be very careful when talking about their own contemplative experience.

One of the main rediscoverers of that tradition, in our Canadian context, was the Benedictine Dom John Main, who moved into this house and began to teach this form of Christian contemplative prayer, calling it simply Christian meditation. He was helping people who were already into Transcendental Meditation, or who were going to yoga centers or Buddhist meditation centers, to root that meditation practice in the soil of the Christian faith. That's the tradition that we're carrying on as part of our program in this house.

PD: When we talk of traditional medical treatment and healing, I think everyone now recognizes that technology is so far ahead of our ability to bring values and ethics to the practice, that we're able to do things now without knowing whether we should do them. The kind of healing you're working on is simpler, is within all of us, isn't it?

TR: Yes. I think the religious journey is not a question of becoming something other than what we are, but of becoming more aware of who we already are and living that fully. So at the heart of our own human vocation is a mystical experience. At the root of our human existence, we are always and everywhere held in existence by a compassionate, loving Presence who is present to us more deeply than the beat of our own hearts and the lifeblood coursing through our own jugular.

Coming to an awareness of that and living more fully in that awareness is the quintessential religious experience. That is what we as Christian churches have to learn from the Eastern religions. The primary business of religion is to provide an experience of God, to provide people with an experience of that Presence that dwells within them.

Chapter 7
ENERGY FOR CHANGE

The Healing Power of Anger

Kathryn
McMorrow

❧

ی

Twenty years ago, I suffered from panic attacks. To this day, I vividly remember how they could descend like a surprise thunderstorm in the summer and vanish as quickly as a rainbow. One particular incident landed me in the emergency room of a suburban Montreal hospital. Once this "storm" had passed, and wanting to apologize for wasting his time, I rather sheepishly said to the doctor, "I guess it's just in my head." His response was as perceptive – remember this was over 20-odd years ago – as mine was wrong. He said, "Nothing is ever 'just' in your head."

Today of course, no one would dispute the vital bridge between our physical and emotional states – there's a virtual traffic jam of signals crossing that link. After our mind draws the broad outlines of our life, the colors are born from our emotional palette. One of the darkest is anger – a protean bully that can, one day, keep us from making a connection, while preventing us from letting go of one the next.

I think we all know how anger can be the nastiest and most stubborn roadblock on the journey to any destination, but especially so when we're striving for wellness and balance in our lives. Kathryn McMorrow offers a way to actually use all that energy from anger to arrive at forgiveness and healing, and ultimately, to change the colors of our life "picture." Professionally, she has a Master's degree in teaching and one in clinical psychology. Of equal importance, she is, in person, warm and friendly, with the rare gift of being a good listener.

Ms. McMorrow lives at Unitas, the ecumenical center for spirituality and Christian meditation in Montreal.

ی

KM: Unitas is something that I've been involved with for about four years and it's very dear to my heart.

PD: Why is it so dear to your heart?

KM: Because of its philosophy. The mission statement of Unitas is something that I firmly believe in. It gives me a chance to empower other people, to offer a healing environment, right downtown, where people can come no matter what their financial situation.

I don't own many possessions, but I certainly appreciate beautiful surroundings. To think that one family with four children lived in this wonderful house and now it's available to hundreds of people, it's something that's very much a mission statement for myself and my life.

I've also, like many other people, faced anger issues in my life. The fact that I've done a lot of my own healing around that makes me want to provide a space where other people can do the same.

PD: I was saying to Father Ryan that I think if you had to identify the emotion bubbling just under the surface of this world it would be anger. But I wonder if part of the problem is getting people to identify it as anger. Why is that so hard?

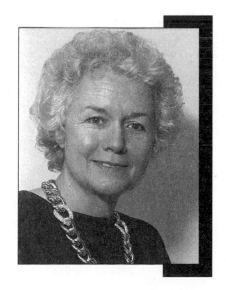

KM: Well, it is hard. I give workshops in a one-day format, or on two Wednesday evenings in a row. People come in on the first Wednesday and I go through an instructional model with them. The homework is to get angry during the week. Now, most people don't have any problem with that, they like those assignments! What's interesting, though, is that people will come back the next Wednesday and I know they will say to me, "You know, I wasn't as angry as I was last week," or "I started to get angry and then I started wondering what the feeling was underneath." The very fact of becoming aware changes our behavior.

I firmly believe that to live fully and to develop our spirituality we have to have a sense of who we are. To have a relationship with God or the Goddess or the sacred – however you conceptualize that – we have to bring a sense of self to that; it has to be a real I/thou relationship, to quote Martin Buber. A lot of what prevents us from finding out who we are is a layer of anger.

So in the workshop, I start by asking, "What does it mean to be human?" To be human is to have needs. You can use any number of models to talk about this. Maslow's hierarchy of needs is an easy one. If people have never seen it before, it's an easy one to catch on to quickly. If they have seen it before, I explore different ways of looking at it.

So we have needs as human beings and we also have basic human rights. That always opens up discussion too: Do we really have human rights? Does a person have a right to exist because they're human? The United Nations Charter of Rights says we do. We live in a country where we recognize human rights, where I can actually say something out loud and not be afraid of going to prison. A lot of people who maybe haven't traveled much take these things for granted. Sometimes, it's the first time in people's lives they've really thought about what this means.

Now, when those needs and rights are being threatened or abused, my body takes on a very natural, healthy, lifesaving response; I become angry. But before I become angry, I become fearful. It's a way of protecting myself and of doing something about what I'm afraid of, or about what's threatening me. That's why we call anger a secondary emotion. Often, people aren't in touch with the needs or the rights that are being abused; they only know they are angry. To say, "I need something," or "I'm afraid of something," is difficult for both men and women. We're not socialized to actually talk about that or to feel vulnerable.

I don't like to generalize, but, quite often, men have been socialized to think that it's okay to show anger, but not to show vulnerability, hurt, or insecurity. For women, sometimes, it's okay to cry and it's okay to look helpless and all that stuff, but don't get angry.

So when people come to the anger workshop, some people need to get angry in order to make changes, because the energy is in the anger. That's the point at which anger can be good.

PD: So you use it to reach a state of healing?

KM: Absolutely. When it comes to healing, though, the other thing I have to mention is expectations. We grow up with expectations of ourselves and others have expectations of us too. Perfectionism produces a lot of anger.

So very gently, in the workshop, we recognize our needs and our rights. When I first start the workshop I say, "Think of a situation recently, or from way back, when you've been angry and it's still living with you."

And they take that anger that they're feeling and they

go back and they say, "Okay, what need was being abused here?" I give out a list of rights and needs; we look at Maslow's hierarchy here. What need was not being met? What was I afraid of? Quite often, people go out of the workshop saying, "I'm not afraid of my anger anymore because I know where it's coming from."

PD: Maslow's hierarchy is...?

KM: Basically, Maslow said that we have a variety of needs that form a kind of hierarchy. It helps to think of this as a pyramid. The first level, or the base of the pyramid, is made up of our physiological needs. We need air to breathe, food to eat, water to drink, and so on. The second level, moving up the pyramid, is made up of safety and security needs. We need shelter, for example. The third level is made up of belonging and love needs. We need to feel as though we're part of a larger group of people, of a community. The fourth level is made up of esteem needs. We need a sense of achievement and recognition. The fifth level is made up of cognitive needs. We need knowledge and understanding. The sixth level is made up of aesthetic needs. We desire order and beauty. And at the very top of the pyramid, is our need for self-actualization. We need to realize our potential.

A critical part of Maslow's theory is that we must satisfy, at least to a significant degree, a need which is lower on the pyramid before we can move to the need above it. So we need to have air and food and water before we can start to think about shelter. And once we have our shelter needs met, we can begin to think about our need for other people. And once we have a place in the community, we can begin to think about our esteem needs and what we have to contribute, and so on, all the way up the pyramid.

Now, in the anger workshops, I take some of this theory and apply it to the experience of the child, because a lot of the anger that people are carrying is from childhood.

And I say, "Okay, when a baby comes into the world, what does it need?" Well, it needs to be fed, it needs to be held. A lot of very deep-seated anger is being carried from this period of life because some of these needs were not met. People will sometimes say, "I don't have any words for this anger." Well, maybe it goes back to a time when they didn't have any words, when the child couldn't express itself verbally.

People are always asking me, can you go back to your birth and relive it? I have never personally lived that kind of experience. I know professionals who do that kind of work and there are people in the workshop who will say, "I went back and I experienced something when I was six months old." If you experienced it, it's legitimate.

PD: Is anger ever anger, just for or by itself?

KM: A lot of anger comes from the past, but there's enough stress out there and enough shortages and enough people not respecting each other that I can be very legitimately angry in the here and now.

But anger for itself is always the result of one of my rights being abused or threatened, or one of my needs not being met. Or of having expectations – of myself or of others – that are too high. Somebody's being rude to me, somebody cuts me off on the expressway. If I recognize the source of the anger, express it appropriately in the here and now, and let it go...

PD: That's okay, it's legitimate?

KM: It's finished, it's legitimate.

I have a whole list of words that we go through: the difference between anger, aggression, hostility, frustration. You see, anger is the emotion, pure and simple. Aggression is the behavioral component of anger and some people only know anger and aggression together. For them, to get angry means to hit somebody, or to see somebody angry means to get hit by somebody. Or it's the boss, which means power and control are involved.

People learn that when they're angry, they have choices. They can have a temper tantrum if they want, but is this serving them or is it not? Is it respectful of other people or is it not? Our bodies prepare, physiologically, to fight or flee with anger – that's why it's so hard on our systems when we keep carrying it.

The other word we look at is resentment which in French – ressentiment – is to feel it over and over and over again. If I resent somebody else for 20 years, I am putting myself through this anger thing and it's not going anywhere. The only person it's hurting is me: my health, my relationships. I'm holding on to the past, I'm keeping a relationship with this person.

People ask, "What's the opposite to love?" A lot of people say hate. But the opposite of love isn't hate, it's indifference. So if I still hate somebody, I'm holding on to that relationship, I'm connecting, it's still important. I mean, some people like the hate relationship better than the love relationship!

PD: How do you deal with anger that comes from hurt, not from fear? People can be so badly hurt by life.

KM: The first step is to recognize and express the anger. In the case of a husband losing his wife, it's not only the death, it's the loss of his whole plan for the future. And then it's all caught up with, "Well how can I be mad because my wife has died? My kids are without a mother..." Who's he going to get angry at, how's he going to do that? It's not easy.

Then you need to live the pain. When people are angry all their lives, it's often because of fear; they do not want to live the pain.

The pain of actually admitting and accepting anger needs to be handled in therapy sometimes. If there are deep, deep hurts, it sometimes requires that someone be there with you, to journey with you. Other times, they can do it in the forgiveness workshop, or they can come to this house for some private time to heal.

People have been meditating here for 15 years so the vibrations... People come in and say the silence isn't empty here, there's a fullness here in the silence. So they feel that it's a safe place.

In the workshop, one of the first things I create is safety around just what the workshop is and isn't going to be. We're respectful of each other. We're here to do our own stuff, and when we do partner work, it involves active listening. I'm not going to tell you what to do and I'm not going to comment on how you shouldn't feel that way. Healing takes place because someone says, "Hey, here's a new way of being and I have the right to that. I can do it."

PD: Is there a physical way to come to terms with anger, to deal with it?

KM: When I get angry, the energy is there for me to do something about it. You know, it's either fight or flee. But how do you do that in a boardroom? How do you do that when you've got small children to raise? You've got all this energy going – the heart beating, the muscles tensing, adrenaline shooting into your system. Adrenaline is a very powerful hormone, a very powerful drug. You can get addicted to adrenaline.

One of the things I ask the group is: "What are the advantages of being angry? What is the payoff? How do you feel when you're angry?"

Maybe, for the moment, you feel powerful, but afterward, you feel like a jerk! So if you recognize that, then we say, "Okay, can you do something else that will give you that amount of satisfaction and not have the negative side effects?"

One of the things in dealing with anger is how do you calm yourself down enough so that you can hold on to enough energy to go after what you need. One of the problems is that people say, "Just calm down." But by the time you've calmed down, you say, "Oh well, I guess it wasn't that bad and I guess he didn't really mean what he said and I guess my kid is okay." Until the next time, when you go through the whole thing again.

So we brainstorm how to do it for each person. And it's different for each person. And then we explore how to state your needs. It's the whole assertive thing. Describe what you need, state the consequences, how you felt. We have a lot of fun with that because we do role plays. For example, how do you tell someone how you feel, objectively, without calling them a jerk?

PD: It's impossible!

KM: It's not, Peter! Peter, it's not! Believe me, if I can do it anybody can do it!

PD: But in that moment of anger, it's virtually impossible to step back.

KM: That's right. But I always say to people who come to a workshop, "You're all here because you've been handling anger. None of you is behind bars, you're running your own lives. That means you've been able to do it so far. You're here because you want to find some ways that work better."

It can be a small thing, something that takes a matter of seconds. For example, when you're sitting in a boardroom, just pull your chair back, get some space between you, because when you're angry you lean toward the person. Or have a glass of water. Do anything for those few seconds to break the cycle.

Sometimes people will come back the next week and say, "I did some of these techniques, otherwise I would have killed that person," so to speak. What happens with your brain when you're under stress is that your thinking gets distorted. That's why we do things when we're angry that afterward cause us to say, "What happened to me?"

So I pull back and breathe; that's what I use all the time, the breathing. You let your system calm down. It's not a case of taking ten breaths so I can be patient. It's so my whole system can calm down, so I can see a little more clearly. Quite often, it's simply a matter of not responding at the moment.

PD: Would you concede that sometimes the expression of anger is really and truly satisfying?

KM: Sometimes, Peter.

PD: I mean sometimes you know, in the middle of it, that you're being a jerk. But there are other times when you think that the person deserves more than you can possibly say or do at that moment!

KM: Exactly.

PD: So is that kind of anger an obstacle to healing?

KM: I guess you need to ask yourself what the outcome is going to be and whether or not you're respecting the other human being.

The other word we discuss is rage and that refers to the intensity of anger, when something has been done that has really been hurtful and has been a betrayal – that sort of thing.

Sometimes the amount of anger is commensurate to the act. But often I'm carrying this whole gunny sack of anger from childhood and all the stuff I haven't expressed. Then I've got the whole day on my shoulders and some poor soul toward the end of the day happens to say or do something, and I not only give him or her what they deserve, but I give them a little bit of everything I've been carrying around with me. That's the hard part of it.

But when someone is doing something that's totally un-acceptable as a human being, the rage on the part of the person can be very appropriate and the intensity of the anger can send the message, "This is how strongly I feel about this."

For myself, I do not believe that violence is appropriate in any shape or form at any time. That's my own personal feeling and it extends to children and the issue of disciplin-ing them physically. I always ask parents, "If you were calm and cooled down, would you have hit your child that way?"

You may feel like you're in control, but when you think about the times you were most angry, it is usually when you were most out of control. We have a right to our personal space and we need to have personal power, we need to be able to control our own environment. And usually, our anger is greatest when that need is threatened. Using the example of the parent again, if you go back to look at your parents who maybe were yelling at you, for example, those were the times usually when the parent felt, "This kid is driving me nuts. I don't know what else to do!" And yet as children, we didn't perceive it that way. We experienced it as this all-powerful godlike person who was coming down on us.

PD: It's also learned, though, isn't it? If you watched your parents deal with things in an angry way, then that becomes your method of handling life.

KM: In one of the first parts of the session, I give out a page of questions: How did you learn about anger? What did your mother teach you about it? How did your parents show it to each other?

Depending on what the needs in the group are, somebody will usually say that was the part that really made it clear to them. We do that, first, individually, and take some quiet time for reflection.

Then, when we come together in a group. I usually ask, "Who in here had a good, strong, healthy role model?" I do this because, often, people feel guilty or they think there's something wrong with them because they're coming to look at this and having trouble with it. And I point out to them that I have yet to meet somebody who says their parents expressed anger well.

Often, they will say, "Oh no, my parents never got angry!" Or they say, "Oh no, they never had an angry word between them!"

In those instances, I figure that one of the parents was living their life and the other was following along, or that we will discover that one of them had a heart attack at 48, or that someone will say, "My mother had migraines all the time, but she never got angry."

PD: I'm guessing you see and hear this all the time with couples who have been together ten, 15, or 20 years, that some anger is bubbling just under the surface. It's recognized by the couple as anger, but they feel helpless in the face of it, to deal with it in a healthy way. It seems to be a constant wound.

KM: Because they've never learned how to deal with it. Now I don't know what the marriage encounters are offering these days, but there's probably a component of conflict resolution in them. Just the idea that there is going to be conflict and it is going to be healthy is often new for couples. If there's no conflict, you're going to bore each other to death. But what do we do about the conflict?

I think there's a whole new mind set around that and what excites me – because I do work in schools, I taught human sexuality and personal social education for many years and I train teachers in that – is that kids are learning about this in elementary school and parts of these programs deal with conflict resolution and communication skills. I always ask people who come to the workshops, even those in their early 20s, if they have ever had any courses in conflict resolution, in communication skills, or in active listening. Nobody.

Well, if the school is really putting that program in place and is serious about it and they've got good teachers doing it, kids are now going to learn this.

PD: It seems like this course should be part of the fundamentals.

KM: Absolutely.

PD: But in the West, at least, we live in such a competitive environment, whether it's business or personal, it's quite amazing we don't pay more attention to it.

KM: But kids are doing it, again, in schools where they're using collaborative learning, where people work in teams. They have their own things to do, but they also help each other. I have a lot of hope for the way children are growing up. Having said that, however, the family unit – whoever is at home – still has an extremely powerful influence on these kids, especially during the first few years of life.

But the word is influence. It's not like I'm condemned to behave forever in a certain way. It explains where my behavior comes from. But now, as an adult, I have a choice.

PD: We know the rituals of anger much better than we know the rituals of healing, don't we?

KM: It seems that way. And the ritual of healing is so personal. But it happens when I can recognize the anger and go into the pain and know that it takes time. When I do the forgiveness workshop, we look at forgiveness as a process, not as an event.

It's a wonderful workshop because we get rid of all the myths. For instance, forgiveness is not a moral obligation. It is a choice. It is an act of the will. It is a choice to enter into the process, which means I'm going to have to look at the anger and I'm going to have to look at the pain. One of the myths is that, if I forgive the person, I have to have a relationship with them. It doesn't mean that at all.

Also, what drives people nuts are those who go around forgiving people for everything. I'm five minutes late and so the person says, "I forgive you!" Talk about anger! There are certain things that are appropriate, although very difficult, to forgive: betrayal, deep betrayal of a person in a relationship; brutality; disloyalty.

Some people, because the pain is so strong, have trouble actually admitting what was done to them. They – a woman who is being beaten, or a person who is living with an alcoholic or a drug addict – will make all kinds of excuses for the other person. So another thing we say about forgiving is that you don't do it if the behavior is continuing. That's co-dependency, that's hurting yourself.

PD: Forgiveness has to be given from a point of emotional and physical safety. But it takes courage to do that, to offer your heart, in effect, to someone and to say here it is. You leave yourself in a very vulnerable position. But I suppose it makes you stronger.

KM: Peter, that's it. What power that implies! What that says is, "I care for myself enough, I feel that I am enough of a person to forgive so that I can move on." To forgive is not to condone. We forgive for ourselves, so that we can live in the future. We forgive so that we can recognize that we're human and that the other person is human, and that we're not judging or condoning their behavior.

That was one of the hardest things for me because I thought, if I forgive that person, it's like I'm saying, okay, keep doing it! You can forgive someone and still take them to court. They're still responsible for their behavior, but you can let go of the anger, the resentment. Forgiveness often has nothing to do with the other person.

And you're right, it is saying, "Yes, I was vulnerable and I was hurt, but I want to move on and to be open to other people."

PD: But in that process of healing, it almost seems to me that forgiving yourself is harder.

KM: That's what comes out in the workshop. We ask people, "Who would you like to forgive?" Often, the answer comes back, "I'd like to forgive myself." How could I have been so stupid as to get into that relationship? Why didn't I think of everything at once? Why did I let that go on so long? Why wasn't I perfect? Why wasn't I godlike?

To forgive yourself is to live the pain of not being perfect, of not being totally aware. It is to accept that imperfection and then to ask what did I learn out of that? What's going to change? Forgiveness involves a paradigm change. You move out of your old way of thinking and into another paradigm. I think that's what we're moving toward in the 21st century. I think it was Einstein who said, "You don't solve a problem within the same paradigm."

PD: Right.

KM: But that's what we keep trying to do!

PD: But it's got to be more than a temporary shift.

KM: Yes. We have to live out of it from now on. When I get angry, I'm going to look at what my needs are, what my rights are, and I'm not going to wait for 20 years or even, perhaps, two days.

PD: So are you healing the same person or becoming someone new? Or does that distinction even matter?

KM: I think it matters incredibly. I think we're becoming a new person with every instant. And also, I really believe that I'm a part of all that I've met. I teach counseling skills at McGill and people will say, "Well, if I didn't help them, at least I didn't hurt them." Not true. You will change any person you come into contact with in some way or another. It's either going to be in a way that empowers them – you address the person at Maslow's level of self-actualization, creativity, and the development of who they are – or they're going to feel diminished in some way as a result of your interaction with them.

PD: What's the spiritual price we pay for not dealing with anger?

KM: The age of depression might be a good phrase, or the age of anxiety. The spiritual price we pay is not becoming who we are meant to be or who we really are. It's not so much a case of actively striving toward this true self as it is a matter of letting go of this anger so that this incredible person can come out and be who he or she is. It's a very high price that we pay. We pay it in relationships, we pay it in our health, we pay it in our creativity and where we want to go. So, for me, it's almost the price of being human. We really prevent our humanity from coming out. It's an incredible price.

PD: I wonder how we've arrived at a point where we're so afraid to be who we are? Do you understand why we add layers on or build walls around who we are? Father Ryan spoke about how this house is about finding out who you are and about then being comfortable with what you find.

KM: Well, I tend to think we're becoming a lot closer to who we are. For example, one of the reasons I'm giving this type of workshop is because it wasn't around when I needed it.

When we talk about anger, there are times when we can't address the source of our anger directly, but we can address it in other ways. For example, one of the things I did last year was to create a workshop on incest and sexual abuse for non-therapists, as an education tool. That was my anger energy, which grew from my recognition of a serious social problem, going into that. It's an energy for change, it's an energy that says, "I don't like what's going on right now and I want to do something about it!" So I'm probably more angry in some ways than I used to be because I'm more in touch. But it's a positive energy which motivates me to make some changes.

I wanted a place like Unitas to exist so I give a tremendous amount of my time for that to happen. But the satisfaction I get out of it is incredible. The important thing about this house is that each person that's here has certain gifts and certain qualities, and when those are honored and allowed to find expression, the synergy is incredible. There's an energy for change! I really believe, Peter, that we are developing more as human beings.

PD: This is less flippant than it may sound, but how do you know when you've found who you are?

KM: I think probably we have that feeling without really identifying it as "who we are." And now this sounds like a paradox, but it has to do with transcendence, which is something Maslow added after talking about self-actualization. We become aware of and get in touch with everyone and everything around us.

I often ask people, "When are you not aware of the time passing? When are you are so taken with something that your entire self is put into that? When do you live out of your qualities or gifts so that the energy is just flowing?" At those times, you can say the Holy Spirit is moving in me, or you can say I'm in touch with universal energy, but you feel good about what you're doing.

It's not mood altering and that's an important point because one of the ways of handling anger is to become addicted – and you can be addicted to anything. To lift up an addiction is to look at pain.

So when I'm not addictive, when I'm not mood altering, when I'm simply getting high on being who I am, people get annoyed and sometimes say, "Kathryn, what are you so happy about? Where do you get off being so happy?"

Because I paid my dues, number one. I've done a lot of my healing, though I know I still have some to do.

And I'll ask people, "When were you awake today? What really got you excited?" And they'll respond, "Well, it was when I was helping that kid," or "It was when I was doing that painting." That is when you're in touch with who you are.

It's not the intention that I do these things so that other people will benefit, but I believe that when we're in touch with our gifts and are living them, other people do benefit. I think that's a universal law. But it comes out of who I am rather than out of a decision to do this particular thing.

It's very empowering for me to know that there's a difference happening with people. We sat in this room on Sunday and people grieved, and the forgiveness... They went out feeling, "Yea, I'm in the process and I'm ready to go further and I want to have a life."

PD: So you see people's tears as much as their anger?

KM: Oh yes. People often ask, "Aren't you worried about those who come to this anger workshop?" It's not the ones who come that worry me, it's the ones out there who don't come, or the ones who say to the ones who come, "I'm glad you're going to that workshop. You sure need it!" Those are the ones I worry about.

But it's incredible. When someone comes to an anger workshop, they're actually saying, I want to take responsibility for this. I tell people that when they come to a workshop, most of the work is over. They come when they're ready to come and that's why they're so successful.

PD: You have to be ready to heal.

KM: Yes, and you've done a lot of the work because you're coming. I'm very fortunate that in almost all of my work, people come to the workshops because they want to. In the hospital where I'm going tomorrow, the staff asked for it, they wanted it, and they're all coming. The motivation is there and the desire is there.

PD: There's always much talk around the end of a millennium, but it does seem to me to be true that the rate of change has been so extraordinary for all of us, at the end of this century, that it must contribute to feelings of anger and unease.

KM: Yes. David Elkind wrote *The Hurried Child* 20 years ago, and Toffler, in *Future Shock*, was pleading with us to slow down.

Corporations and institutions, ethically, have to really look at this. People are constantly being put into a fight or flight response because they're being forced to adapt so fast and they're worried about what the next adaptation is going to be. The group I'm working with on Friday wants to know how to motivate employees during times of change. It's probably one of the most difficult things to do.

I point out that, the more I identify with my outside roles rather than with who I am, the harder it is. If I'm really in touch with who I am, I'm going to make decisions out of who I am. And so I may resist the change, or I may go with it, but I will adapt to it.

There's still this idea that there's something innately good about change. Not so. I can go through several seeming changes, but the center and core of who I am does not change.

PD: But that stress fuels impatience. We want cures more than healing.

KM: Often, people will ask two things. First, "How long is this going to take?" I can't really answer that for somebody else. It may take a long time. But you have to realize that once you're in the process, you can choose what to focus on. You can choose to focus on the ten minutes or two hours today when you were unhappy, or you can choose to focus on what went well.

We used to have, in the Catholic tradition, an examination of conscience at the end of the day. Just before you went to sleep, you were to go through all the things you did wrong. What a way to end the day!

When I was going through my own personal healing, one of the counselors said to make it, at the end of the day, an examination of consciousness. When was I awake? When was I in touch with my gifts? What situations did I handle well? When did I manage my anger well this week?

The tendency is to move toward whatever you focus on. So why not focus on what you did well?

The other question people ask is, "Can I ever heal completely from this particular thing?" My tendency would be to say, if the person asking the question is in my workshop, "Yes, you can." The fact that they have come to the workshop and are able to structure, from a psychological point of view, their way in the world, means, I believe, that they have enough self-esteem to do an incredible amount of work.

You know some of these books that say, "It's never too late to have a happy childhood"? Well, if my childhood wasn't happy, all the pretending in the world is not going to change that. What I need to do is go back and grieve not having a happy childhood.

As a child, I'm totally dependent on other people for my self-esteem, but as an adult, I'm not. And that makes a big difference when it comes to healing. As an adult, I don't have to depend on you or on anybody else for my value. And for some people, just recognizing that truth is the major step.

So how do I heal? By continuing to explore these questions: What are my gifts? How am I going to protect those? How am I going to behave in a way that's respectful of myself and others? That's healing, Peter. That's healing because I've changed and because I've deepened my awareness of who I am.

Chapter 8

HEAR THE CRIES

The Healing Community *Barbara Bishop*

❧

*"...if all we do is dream about what ought to be,
and never seriously address what is,
God is not set free to transform us..."*

*A few words from a 1993 sermon which define the very nature
and intention of Barbara Bishop's determined ministry. Reverend Bishop delivered this sermon to her congregation at Woodbine Heights Baptist Church in Toronto after ten months experience with a national pilot project called "Fire in the Rose," dedicated to exploring and addressing family violence.*

*As you're about to discover, it was precisely an incident of
abuse which brought Barbara Bishop to the pulpit, and she stands
there neither easily nor is much concerned with offering soothing
platitudes for her congregation. Upon meeting her in person,
one realizes quickly how dedicated she is to making a difference
in the so-called "real" world, and how much her heart aches
from the stories of abuse to be found there. She is uncomfortable
with the label of "healer," but it is an accurate one, as her heart
embraces hurt, shares the pain, and in the end, confirms the
value and importance of community and caring.*

*"...we ask God to do the forgiving, for we are outraged,
blind with grief, torn apart by feeling our brothers'
and sisters' suffering. It is enough.
God will take us all from there..."*

❧

PD: How did you come to the ministry?

BB: It was about 15 years ago, I guess. I was a teacher. I was a deacon in our church, and I was a very active lay woman. There was a woman in the congregation who was withdrawing from life, from us, and I asked the minister about it. He said, "Go visit her." So I did.

She told this story, and in the process of working through, first, my shock that the guy who takes up the offering is beating his wife (this type of thing is very difficult for most good Christians to accept) and second, what she needed and what we could offer her, I did what I always do. I went to the library. I researched. I looked it up. I learned. I studied. I'm a perpetual student. I felt that what we were doing was wrong, that what the church was doing was contrary to everything that people who were working with these women said would help.

PD: What was the church doing then?

BB: It was trying to mediate. It's very common that the male minister, with all good intentions, will sit down with the couple and tell them to lighten up, like let's work this thing out. But what would happen then, in the course of the interview, is that the male batterer would perceive the male pastor as being an ally. The woman would go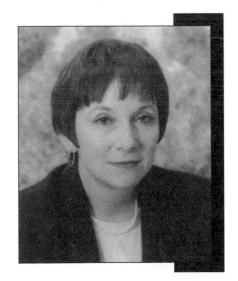

home and she would be accountable for anything that she said. (When I say "she," I'm speaking generically.) So she would know enough to be quiet and not say too much because it was very dangerous. So a lot of damage was done.

The church has idealized the family in that way, it's like an icon. We worship this whole family value stuff, so preserving the family was perceived as so important...

PD: Almost at any cost...

BB: Oh yes. The dissatisfaction I experience is a growing edge which I think is helpful for me. I feel that if I ever get really satisfied with the church, then I can't do the border-region kind of ministry that I think people are crying for.

PD: What happened in that case you described? What did you do when you realized the church was working against what was probably best for that woman?

BB: I went to seminary. I quit my job. I left teaching after 15 years. I think there were a number of reasons why I did that.

PD: You mean why you went to seminary?

BB: Yes. This was one of the precipitating events that propelled me there. I went to learn and spent my three years working through a whole lot of issues. I did my thesis on pastoral theology of battered women. My issue, interestingly, was not pastoral care – that was kind of instinctive – it was pastoral theology.

For myself, I've always wanted to know, "What are we doing? Why are we doing it? What does it mean?" I have to know what it means. And I think a lot of people who have been hurt as children have a drive, a strong need to understand where reality really is, because we didn't learn it appropriately. So we're detectives. Some survivors become crusaders, they want to make the world right. For myself, I have to understand this; this has to make some sense to me.

So I did this pastoral theology work and integrated feminist theology and sociology and pastoral counseling and put it together in a thesis.

PD: It's really a "whole life" view that you were looking at?

BB: Yes, and I'm always doing that. Wholeness is so important to me, integrity is so important to me. And the reason I like doing what I'm doing right now, though it is very demanding and very stressful, is because it makes sense to me. This is what I should be doing.

It didn't make sense to me to be a minister who sort of preached and prayed and visited and chaired meetings, who had this other passion. But now that I can work it together in the church, everything we're doing here makes sense to me.

Theologically, I suppose, our church is constantly moving in the direction I'm leading, which is scary. You do, as a minister, have a great deal of trust conferred on you, and one of the primary pieces of trust is that you're going to help them make sense of their experience too. So we're all moving together in this.

PD: But all of this made sense to you as much as a survivor of abuse as a minister of the church?

BB: Yes. It would be appropriate to say that early life

experiences in a rural Nova Scotian environment certainly made me alive to those kinds of issues.

PD: So you started with that one specific case, but you've really gone on, haven't you?

BB: The project that we started, "Fire in the Rose," was begun as an educational project. It was financed by Health and Welfare Canada, the Donner Foundation, and it was ecumenical. Can a local congregation make a difference? Can we be educated? Can we learn? From that educational process, in effect, I came out. It gave me permission to use my strengths in ministry. And I was struggling with a way to use my strengths in ministry openly, because I knew that I had, what's the word I'm looking for... I'm resisting the word "gift"...

PD: An ability?

BB: Yes. Since I've been in ministry, people have said that they find me reassuring, they find me healing, they find me helpful. That astonishes me, you know, when they tell me that, but that is consistent feedback. So how to use this in a way that was also prophetic or truth telling, because I didn't want to be just a soother. I didn't just want to be ointment on wounds, though I think that's important.

I've always felt that the truth is what makes us free and that we have to understand what's really happening in our lives. Now, I think most ministers experience this schizoid thing: people walk into your office and you know their real lives and you go out there Sunday morning and take part in worship that lies about everything that's really happening to them.

PD: Be happy with your life now?

BB: Be happy, yea. And it involves triumphalist thinking. Let's claim the victory, victory over the grave, saved from our sins, Jesus has the power, smile, be nice, don't be angry...

PD: What role does truth play in healing, have you come to understand?

BB: Huge. I've come to think that the first thing, the most important thing for survivors of trauma – whether it's abuse or the war or a mugging or whatever – the first thing is safety. And so the first thing that this project allowed me to do was to work with the people here. (I haven't done it alone, I'm very communal in my approach.) It has allowed me to work with them to make the church a safer place for people to be. And people know. As soon as they walk in here, without knowing about "Fire in the Rose" or abuse or survivors or anything, they walk in and they... breathe, and they say, "I can be myself here. This is okay." They just know.
     I like that.

PD: I read recently someone who said that healing is really getting rid of everything that isn't you.

BB: That's a wonderful observation! And so I think as we become more authentic people, then our faith obviously has a whole lot more meaning. Church becomes a safer place because being a safe place as a church means being safe people, not expecting other people to be some kind of Christian clone. Once that safety is in place, then the truth will come out. A survivor said to me once, "It feels like there's so much in my head and the holes aren't big enough for it to come out." I thought that was a powerful statement.

It doesn't even have to be truth about abuse. Maybe the truth is that my husband and I don't get along sometimes. Maybe the truth is that my daughter drives me crazy sometimes. Maybe the truth is that I forgot to make this announcement and I really screwed up and I'm sorry. Maybe the truth is, yea, I shouldn't have said that, you're right. Maybe the truth is, okay, I'll change my mind.

PD: But that can only come with a sense of personal safety?

BB: Yes.

PD: How do you do this?

BB: Well, we have different groups. We have a Bible study called "Square One" which was founded on the theory that anybody can ask anything, as though you're at square one. You can start by asking, "Is there a God?" and "Why?" and "What kind?" We've developed an inquiring, exploratory mode of studying the Bible, and that creates safety.

I preach sermons that come at things from a different perspective, and so those sermons create safety.

Our kids' programs create safety for children and for parents. When people come for kids' programs, we tell them we're aware that they're concerned, in this age, about their children's safety from abuse and that, insofar as possible, we promise to try to look after that. We have committees working on protocols. What would happen if somebody accused somebody else?

We watch the music we use. We do not use violent

music. We try very hard never to use faith to enact violence on people in any way. So I don't march for Jesus. I mean, they can go ahead and march for Jesus, but the image is abhorrent to me. We work very hard on all kinds of peacemaking issues in the church. My associate is seventh generation Canadian black. She's always reminding us that we haven't even started to make it safe for people who are not white. You know, we're just working all the time to try to do better on that.

Along the way, actually this year, I just started my first survivors group and last night I just started a second one.

PD: And anyone who has been abused in whatever way…

BB: The first group is a generic group. They say generic groups never work and I understand that they are difficult; certainly it's slower work. There are eight of us. My co-facilitator is male, he's also an ordained clergy, a very active Baptist like I am. There's another guy in the group and the rest are female. So because there are only two men, and because the man who leads the group with me is an adult child of an alcoholic, he's very alert. He's done his own work around gender issues as well as his own healing, so I feel very safe having him in the group. We decided we'd try this and see if a mixed-gender group would be good. It has been difficult, but it's also good because these men are there because they were abused too, so it's not an "us against them" thing.

My second group is all female and they've asked that it stay all female because they just don't feel safe with men.

PD: How do you proceed? A victim's rights group is not what you're about?

BB: No. What we're about is to try to create a healing community, to recognize that you got hurt in a relationship and nothing but a relationship can help. You know, healing comes in the community. To create a healing community, the content of what we do is not even terribly important, though we work hard at the content. The content is arrived at by consensus, so...

PD: So the meetings are long...

BB: So the meetings are long! Actually it's not bad, because survivors recognize the issues. So last night, we were talking with the new group and the question that keeps coming up is, "What is normal?" In the first group what kept coming up was anger. "What are we going to do about this?" We had a meeting called "Lies the Abuse Taught Me."

The subject of the meeting is not each person walking through their life. It's not even necessarily sharing the story. That only happens as it's safe. In a therapy group there might be – I'm assuming, I've never been in one – more pressure to come clean, to tell your story. My assumption is that the truth doesn't happen until you're safe. So, first you get safe. And if all that ever happens is you get safe, then you've done a powerful, healing work. If the group moves on to truth telling, that's a plus. But the group can't move to truth telling until everybody in it is safe.

PD: An American psychologist has made the point that there is really nothing beneficial about talking to a group of kids in the inner city about conflict resolution if a gun has gone off beside their heads. He says you first have to "debrief" them, you have to validate that experience.

BB: He's right.

PD: And it sounds as if what you're saying is that listening is also healing. I mean, just the act of listening and not feeling the pressure to talk is a step to be taken.

BB: Yup. In our group, there are three members who consistently have asked for permission to pass and we said from the beginning, "You can come here and you can sit and never open your mouth, that's okay, your presence tells us you're with us." And so these three came back week after week after week, the same thing: they'd say, "Pass," or they'd say, "My week's okay," or "My medication is working," or whatever.

Then, over time, we lost one to the hospital; we're praying mightily for her. Now, the other two have started to talk. But it has been four months. And they're talking, not about the trauma, but about the effects of it. They're saying, "This is what 'it' has done to me, and what I struggle with," and "How can I speak openly when everything I was taught was a lie and I lived with secrets?" And so we talk about that.

PD: How do you characterize the condition that you're trying to heal? I guess it's different with everyone, but are there universal points that keep coming up in a group like this?

BB: I think it varies, but we certainly see the effects of severe trauma – the same thing you'd find if you went over to Sarajevo and worked with kids there. I'm sure it would be the same. I mean, to realize that for a little girl to be in her bed at night and be absolutely unsafe, like he could come anytime, he could do anything he wanted. Mom could be in the next room, but if mom doesn't know...

PD: It's as if she's not there.

BB: Yea. Mom's not there. Mom can't help. So how could you ever trust anybody? For those people, it's the sheer terror. They need more than our group can give them. Our group is a secondary support for them in some ways.

I don't know, I'm still working that one through. I'm still trying to figure out what's best on that one because I don't want to do any harm. You know, if someone feels really safe and starts talking about their being molested and this terrified person is in the group, that may not be helpful.

PD: You have to be careful.

BB: We're very careful on this. So there's everything from sheer terror, to what I think is a longer term problem, which someone in the group named very astutely as "failure to thrive."

PD: That's a really interesting phrase, isn't it?

BB: Yes, "failure to thrive." That's from one of our male members, one who's virtually silent.

I got permission from one of the members to tell you what happened to her through the whole church experience.

PD: Sure.

BB: She came. She liked it. She stayed.

PD: This is to the church...

BB: To the church, just the Sunday morning worship. And

then we had a "Fire in the Rose" sermon and it was called "Healing Through Justice." I did a truth telling sermon. I told some stories from the Bible – the rape of Tamar, the Levite's woman, all these terrible stories – and I said, "You know, don't talk to us about forgiveness, what you need to do is hear." My sermon was about the cries, the cries of Tamar, the cries of the concubine, the cries of the incest survivor. If you can't hear them, don't just try to be kind. Don't try to talk to them about forgiveness. You have to hear them.

It was awful. It was a very difficult sermon to preach and a very powerful service. And at the end of the service, everybody stood around a circle in the church and we all sang *Spirit of Gentleness* together. It was very powerful and we had arranged to have some people available for prayer or comfort or whatever after the service. We also asked that children not be present. So we said, "If anyone is finding this difficult, you can stay and there will be someone here."

We thought all this through. Well, this woman and her daughter stayed and they were both crying. They came in and we spent time and she revealed to me this experience she'd had of sexual abuse with her brother – really horrible. She came and saw me once, then she felt good, so she threw herself into the life of the church.

She overdid it, she burned out, she was having trouble coping at work. She crashed. The doctor put her on antidepressants, she saw a therapist at work through employment counseling, and then she came to our group in the fall and decided that this was what she needed to do. So she's been coming to our group.

She took time off work, she did art, she went down to the beach and she sketched. Creativity is really important for women in healing. In the middle of it all, as she was making tremendous progress and coming to see me once a week, bang! Her father died. So she had to go out west and be there and she wasn't ready. She had been preparing herself for this confrontation, but she wasn't ready. And she just freaked out. I was concerned.

But she did it anyway. They had a family conference, she laid it on the line. And she stayed out there for awhile – continued her sick leave – and came back free of her chronic pain! Survivors of abuse have a tremendous amount of chronic pain.

PD: Physical pain?

BB: Physical pain, chronic back pain. Their bodies are clenched and they have neck pain and back pain. She came back free of the pain, ready to work, and just feeling quite freed up. She continues to be in the group.

While she was away, she called a couple of times; when she panicked, she would call. And by the grace of God, I'm telling you, I called her thinking, I wonder if she's okay, I should give her a call. Her line was busy, or something, and I hung up. And as soon as I hung up, it rang and she was there, just hysterical, saying, "I don't know what I would have done if you hadn't been there." I wept.

You know, you struggle always with where is God, and every so often you think it's okay. Occasionally you get a glimpse that there is this compassionate synchronicity working at the heart of healing, that every so often something just happens that's right. You know, so much happens that's wrong.

PD: What's the lesson you take from this woman's life to understand more deeply the healing process? Is it partly confronting those who have hurt you?

BB: I think the courage to confront the truth, however that works. It's not possible for everybody to do that. Some people would be in danger if they did it. I think the sense of safety, the telling the truth, and the ultimate feeling of reconnection that happens. It doesn't mean, and she'll be the first to say this, that everything's fine. She has a long road to walk. But my sense is that she's feeling better connected with herself, with her own body, with being alone (she lives by herself). I mean, she lost a marriage. Through the things that happened to her, she lost so much.

PD: So if she is still on what you call that "long road," does it mean that healing is a process, that you don't ever arrive at being healed?

BB: Yes, I think so. I'm trying to picture it as all these fiber optic wires of reconnection – now that's a mechanical image. Reconnection is so complex that there is a point at which there's enough that you can go back and live an ordinary life.

PD: Are you reconnecting with yourself or with others?

BB: Both. And with a sense of the sacred, of the Divine, of God. There's a wholeness, there's an integrity that starts to happen.

Of course, there's certain things she'll always have to watch for. She's trying to monitor her need to fix things, her need to make people better, her need to draw a quick conclusion. She's monitoring that, and she still does it all the time.

PD: Do you know how it is that we've become disconnected. What are the forces separating one from another?

BB: I don't know. I sometimes think that happened when we stopped being tribal. I don't know.

PD: But you see, if the statistics are true, there are an awful lot of men sitting there with their wives, sitting with their children seeing these reports, watching news accounts, listening to this stuff, and they're lying to themselves.

BB: Yes.

PD: That's what I can't get over.

BB: The lie is everything. The lie and the secret. Until we get it in our heads that the abuser, the perpetrator, is one of us, and maybe it is us, there can't be any healing. As long as we say, "But he's such a nice guy, he wouldn't do that," or "She must be lying, no man would do that to his daughter," it's very hard.

The Bible is helpful because it tells us that it's always happened, this is not new.

I can't speak for Asian cultures and other faiths, but I think all of us clearly have split body and spirit, and have encouraged that split. Whenever you split body and spirit, women are excluded. Why aren't women allowed at the altar? Because we're unclean. Why are we unclean? One of the researchers on wife assault calls it women as appropriate victims.

I think that split has been damaging to us, to men as well as to women. I think women have done a really good job of discovering the power of community and collective thought, but men can't do that.

My husband and I talk about this a lot. Men can fight it, they can resist it, they can do whatever they want, but the statistics are clear: most of the hurting is being done by men. This is the bottom line. So why is it so hard for men to get together and say, "Let's think about what we're doing here?" Why is their first response, "I'm a good guy, don't dump on me?" When I hear that a mother has murdered her child, my first reaction isn't to say, "I'm a good mother, don't look at me." Rather, my first reaction is to say "Oh God..."

Why can't men do that?

PD: You're somebody who likes, I think, to deal in reality. As you said, you want to know how things work and why they work and what the solution is to problems. I was thinking on the way here that I don't know how many conversations over the years I've had about abuse and about violence, but we just don't seem to get a handle on it: men continue to abuse women, human beings continue to use violence against each other. Is it naive to think that that can ever be truly healed?

BB: I was just getting ready for the Bible study tonight; we're doing parables of the Kingdom. And I was reading about the parable of the wheat and the tares [weeds]. In the biblical story, the enemy sows the weeds and the workers say to the farmer, "Didn't you sow good seed?"

The farmer says, "Yes, an enemy has sown this."

They say, "Well then, let's get rid of it."

And the farmer says, "No, let it grow. I'll harvest it at the end."

The author of the book, Robert Capon, who was reflecting on this story, says that the problem with good people is that we think that we can uproot the evil. We don't realize that as soon as we start actively trying to do that, we end up pulling the wheat up with the weeds, we end up pulling out the good with the bad. In the Kingdom mentality, Jesus appears to be saying that it will grow side-by-side.

I really think there's something about the community, and the healing that has to take place in the community, that means we never will uproot evil. I wish that we would. I would like to think that we would.

I have dreams, and I think the dream of God is that violence and abuse would never happen. I want to believe that that might be so.

PD: Maybe part of it is that the healing has to acknowledge the disease?

BB: Yea, it's there. It's real. It lives beside us. It looks like us. Capon says that in the original Greek of the parable, the word that is used for "weed" describes a weed that looks just like wheat. So the problem is that you can't go in and pull it out because you really don't know, until it bears fruit, what's what. And I think we really don't know what's what. It's in each of us.

I don't know, Peter. I don't know what the answer is. I do know that my children did not suffer as much as I did. I do know, and I believe, that their children will suffer less.

PD: You say that, in the healing community you have at

work here, one of the main attributes or virtues of the group is that you have the freedom simply to listen. I'm not sure what that says about our lives, but I don't think it's complimentary and I wonder if our parents, for example, 40 years ago, would have understood that?

BB: No, they would not have, because a primary virtue of our parents was, "Don't upset anyone." I've been involved in a very difficult controversy in our denomination and I took a public stand on the issue. My mother's perception of that was, "I see you're involved in controversy." And I said to her, "Well, you could say that, or you could say I'm trying to do the right thing." In our parents' minds, you would not try to do the right thing if it would upset anyone. And so if my uncle committed suicide, which he did, we couldn't tell anyone. We had to keep the lid on.

But I also see the extreme opposite of that. I look at the younger people in their 20s and teenagers and so on coming up, and I see this raw and aggressive, almost brutal culture that's coming out – that's not what we wanted either.

All of us Martin Luther King Jr. types are really kind of despairing. We thought we were doing the right thing in taking the lid off, and I still think there's a need for that, but anyway, that's a whole other topic!

PD: Well, in a sense it's not, because it speaks, I guess, to your own discomfort in being labeled a healer because you see the reality of it. You understand how bloody difficult it is to heal people.

BB: Yes. And the reason I think the community piece is so critical is that North America is a very brutal world! Other places are too, but the reality of our lives here is that our kids are consistently not valued. So if we create some kind of microcosm where we say, "Children here are valued, and women here are valued, and men and women here will get on with one another, we will learn to talk to each other," if we can create something approximating the Kingdom in this little place, then it has to be good for people.

You can't fix the world, or at least I can't.

PD: But does your healing, "cure" is the wrong word, what does your healing do to the wounds?

BB: It seems to help the tissue grow over them, I guess. I've always believed that scars are scars. But a scar is better than bleeding, and then once that scar is grown over you say, "Okay, let's get on."

I also think there is something here, there's a sense of the grace of God, that transcends even what we're doing or what I'm doing. There are all kinds of survivors' groups out there, there are all kinds of alternate therapies, there are all kinds of medical solutions, but my place is in ministry, in the ministry of the church. So I also think that's a piece of it.

But it's mysterious to me and I don't believe much in faith healing, I don't believe in miracles very much.

Sometimes people get upset with me because I guess I'm a depressive by nature. I once said to someone that the advantage of being a depressive is that you see the world with such clarity.

PD: You can't be paying attention and not be depressed.

BB: We're not a hand-clapping, chorus-singing congregation, but there is a sense of joy here and I think there is a sense of healing here. People leave worship moved, something in them is touched by what happens here, and I'm continually awed, I'm quite amazed by that. Some people come in and like it.

But my pews are not full! I mean, this is a little church; it seats 250, and on a good Sunday we'll get 80. That discourages me.

PD: So how do you see healing then? What are the signs that healing is taking place?

BB: I think that people have a sense of mutual responsibility for their own lives, for each other, for doing what's right. I have a lot of people here who want to do the right things. We've got a box for a baby that we're trying to look after because the mother is on welfare. We've got a hamper for street kids. We've got the food bank. We've got a real... it's not a navel-gazing thing.

PD: I was just going to say there is a superficial healing that says, "Well, I'll you give ten bucks and I'll go home and I'll feel better because I've done something."

BB: Yes.

PD: But you haven't really. There's a connectedness, I suppose, that must be there.

BB: Yes. I think about this church in terms of James Fowler's stages of faith. I think that when I came I was, and probably I still am, at the fourth stage of integration and self-actualization. I think a lot of people come and go from a sort of stage three formula/conformity faith, into a more exploratory mode. But I also have this sense that we're all moving together into what he calls the public church. At that level, you're able to put paradoxes together, you're able to see the wheat and tares growing together and to realize that maybe you can't pull the whole thing up, and that we're not going to be Gandhi and we're not going to be Christ, but we are going to move a little past where we are. I guess my goals are modest.

PD: What you're saying is, "We're going to be here, we won't be Gandhi or Christ, but we will be here."

BB: Yes.

PD: I remember sitting with the mother of a son who had been abused in Newfoundland, and you could see the church up on the hill from their kitchen window where we were sitting. And she said, "You know, I haven't lost faith in God, but I will never set foot in that building again." In varying degrees, across the country, people have been hurt by the church and it's a particular kind of wound, I think. How do you deal with people who have been wounded by the church?

BB: Actually, that's the most difficult piece for me. Because I'm Baptist and because I'm female and because I was involved in "Fire in the Rose," I'm kind of known. There's a network and people will say, "You know, I've heard about Barbara Bishop, you could call her." I get phone calls whenever something comes out – in my case they're Baptist because that's our denomination. I get phone calls from sobbing, broken women.

PD: Who want to say...

BB: Who want to say, "Not only did this happen to me, but when I took it to my church, it was worse. They hurt me again."

They don't call me to talk about what daddy did. They call me to say, "I didn't know..." It's like there's this release and there's this relief that there's somebody there, who's still in it who's prepared to...

PD: Hear it.

BB: To hear it and to say, "That was bad, that shouldn't have happened, that was wrong." So I get phone calls like that and I get referrals. A woman was referred to me whose whole church gathered to shame, blame, exclude and discredit her, and to support the abuser. She's still a wreck. She's not well. She has not healed. And that's the piece of it that's done her in.

People are powerfully affected by what the church has done, not by the abuse itself as much as by what the church does afterward. They feel so betrayed because, very often, they're very religious women, they bought the whole schtik. They're working hard, they're contributing. Everyone knows that women have propped up the church for generations, and they're in there doing their bit and the people they thought they could trust suddenly look at them blankly, as though they're strangers and lepers.

PD: You must feel anger, as somebody so involved with healing.

BB: Oh, I get furious! Furious!

PD: So is there a healing way to deal with that anger? Your first instinct must be to scream, I would think.

BB: Well, I grieve. I grieve a lot when I'm mad. My grief and my anger are never far apart. I rant and rave a bit. I have a best friend who's also a Baptist minister and I call her and rant and rave. And she calls me when she needs to rant and rave. That really helps a lot. She's my reality check, my mirror, my sister – so she's a real help.

I've tried. I've been the route and I've discovered that, in the end, the old boys gather and they slap one another on the back and they close ranks and you're out there. And so is the woman who got hurt. That's what happens.

I remember thinking, at one time, that I could person-ally deconstruct the whole thing. Well, I can't. I've been very involved in committees where I've been in the jaws of the lion. I've been there, and I've seen what happens, and I can't affect it. I guess it sounds pious, but I say, "Well, in the eyes of God, I just have to do what's right."

For me, what I do is not dependent on the results, and I think this may be a female thing. It's dependent on looking in the mirror and asking, "Can I live with this, with what I'm doing?" My task is to live with myself and ask, "Have I done enough? Is there more I need to do? Should I stop here? Is it time to rest? Was this the right thing to do for her or for him?" That's how I live with it.

My anger at what's happened to these women is huge.

PD: Your energies, at that point, have to go into healing?

BB: Yea. You see, I would be dead if I tried to fight that. I have to protect my own resources so that I can accomplish something. Choose your battles, I guess.

Chapter 9

HOPE AND RISK

The Social Healing of *Lois Wilson*

☙

࿇

Albert Schweitzer was asked once why he would give up his cozy, abundantly comfortable life in Europe to care for the ill and poor in Africa. His response, "I want my life to be my argument," makes me think of the Very Reverend Lois Wilson. Simply put, her life has been consumed by the pursuit of social justice and her efforts to observe, encourage, and report on human rights have taken her in many directions.

In addition to her current duties as chancellor of Lakehead University in Thunder Bay, she is vice president of the Civil Liberties Association of Canada, a panel member of the Public Review Board of Canadian Automobile Workers, and this conversation took place in between her work as a panel member of the Canadian Environmental Assessment Agency reviewing the management and disposal concept of nuclear waste. In the past, she has been moderator of the United Church of Canada and president of the Canadian and World Council of Churches.

What I regret is that, somehow, I've never had a chance to sit down and talk with her until now. I left her company pleased that everything I had heard about her is true. She is smart, tough, funny, unsentimental, determined, passionate, and articulate in her continuing "argument" for social justice and healing around the world and here at home.

࿇

PD: Do you know where that sense of social justice came from in your life?

LW: Oh yes.

PD: It's something that has always been there?

LW: It was in my home. My father was a United Church minister. I came off the prairies and the movement for social justice in Canada came from there. The whole move toward pensions, Medicare, the old Canadian Commonwealth Federation – that was a very strong component. So when you go to Saskatchewan, they take you to see the Credit Union, and, if they've time, you can go and see the Mayor!

And also through the Student Christian Movement where I was very active in my student days. By the age of 18, I understood that my Christian faith had to do with social justice, it had to do with a global perspective, and it had to do with bringing people together in new configurations.

PD: I heard it said recently that the political climate in North America in the last, say, ten to 15 years has made the denial of compassion acceptable. I wonder, as somebody who has fought her whole life for social justice, if that rings a bell with you? Does it sound true to you?

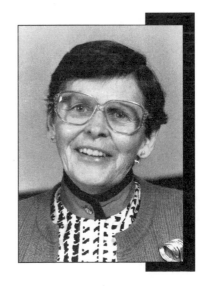

LW: Yes, it does and certainly the whole impetus for social justice is well underground these days.

PD: What's happened to that, do you think?

LW: Well, I wish I knew. What I perceive happening is people putting up, either symbolically or materially, fences and fortresses around themselves, protecting their own financial security.

I mean, in Ontario, you've got banks making record profits and people being cast off their jobs and losing their houses. It's wicked!

PD: So how do you go about – I don't know if this is part of social justice – but how do you go about ever getting one of those bankers and one of those laid off workers to talk with each other?

LW: Well, I think it has larger dimensions than that. It is a societal problem, so you've got to do some social analysis. They may be very nice people. The banker might be a very caring person, but he's in this system, and the same with the person on the street.

So that's why I say my whole ministry has been not so much in terms of individuals, but in terms of the systems we've got out there which prevent people from coming together.

PD: But doesn't systemic change depend initially on individual change or can you attack the system itself?

LW: Not necessarily. It's both/and. You remember, or perhaps you don't, in the Second World War when the U.S. integrated the armed forces and they put Afro-Americans into the army and everybody thought this is going to be terrible. That was a systemic change and pretty soon they found out it wasn't so terrible.

So I think that sometimes the systemic change affects our attitudes as individual initiatives also affect the system. I think they're symbiotic. I'm not prepared to say you've got to have one and then the other. I think that's crazy.

PD: But in trying to understand why it has gone "underground," as you say, economics is number one on your list?

LW: Values. Values are first.

PD: Are people embarrassed to express values publicly now, do you sense?

LW: I think that we once were, but more and more, because we're at such a low ebb, I think that that's going to become more prominent as the situation gets much worse – which it will.

PD: I guess it's been co-opted, in some respects, by politicians to talk of values, especially so-called "family values" south of the border.

LW: Well, I must say that the religious communities have not covered themselves with glory.

PD: Does that come from a fear of appearing judgmental?

LW: Yes, I think so. To be a self-declared Christian in our society is not a popular thing to be. I mean, people aren't very comfortable at all and I'm in situations, because I work a lot in the secular community, where to be known as a Christian minister is still at the level of a funny joke.

PD: So that must affect the work.

LW: They're very uncomfortable until they find out you're a real human being!

PD: I remember speaking with David MacDonald about Stephen Carter's book *The Culture of Disbelief*, and he said the same thing about when he first got to Ottawa. When people found out he was a United Church minister and they were sitting around the Cabinet table, they would be a lot more careful about their language.

LW: Oh yea. Language changes, topics change. It's crazy.

You know, when you asked me before about where the social justice thing had come from, a lot of my early nurture was, as I say, in my home, my church, and the Student Christian Movement. But when I started traveling the globe in 1972, it confirmed many of those earlier convictions.

For example, I went to India and saw people sleeping on the streets. Now I see them in Toronto sleeping on the streets – not in the same numbers, but they're still there. So it was not a shock in the sense that I already knew the problem existed. The experience reconfirmed my convictions.

It was the first time, when I went to India, that I was a minority as a Christian in a sea of Hindus, with some Muslims. So when I got back to Canada I perceived that that was one of the other areas that needed some social healing in our country. Many of the things I discovered when I went on trips abroad confirmed the values I already held.

PD: One of the strongest impressions I left India with was that everyone belonged. It didn't matter if you were living on the sidewalk or on the road, I mean literally living on the street. There was a community there that you belonged to. I sure have the feeling when I pass someone sleeping on a grate here in Toronto or in Montreal, that they've been put aside, they're not in the community anymore.

LW: We've a very individualistic way of looking at things in the West. Asia has more of a communal, interdependent way, which I guess they've had to have.

PD: That must make social healing harder.

LW: Very hard, it's very difficult.

PD: To get to people to say that they have, that there is a responsibility...

LW: Well, and the whole emphasis on individual human rights and me and my family and my income and my children and my place.

PD: How do you spark that "collective" spirit in people?

LW: I'm not really sure. It would be different in different contexts. Sometimes it comes out of tragedy, sometimes it comes out of near tragedy, or when people perceive what's happening and so are motivated to take some positive initiatives.

PD: I remember reading someone who said of Bobby

Kennedy's presidential campaign in the U.S. that his genius was making the rich feel like they were going to be better off if the poor were helped.

LW: Well everybody has to find that they have a stake in what's happening, that in fact that's really what they're meant to have in the community.

When we were in Thunder Bay, the very first thing I did, and I learned a lot from it, was a program we called "Town Talk." It was based somewhat on the American town meeting, but with variations.

One of the things I learned from that is the vocational role of various segments of the community. I mean, the business of "Business" is to do business, to make a profit. That's what business is about. And the schools and universities are to educate; the churches are to raise the moral and ethical issues. And if you get these people, those segments of society in some creative interaction, then they're all winners. They see how they fit into the community and how, if any segment is not doing its job, the whole community is diminished.

PD: How did you do that in Thunder Bay? I was going to ask you about that, I didn't know whether it felt like ancient history to you.

LW: Oh it is ancient history, but it is very much *apropos.*

PD: Because that was back in the 1960s wasn't it?

LW: Yes, it was 1967. It was a communications exercise for the community, to help the community identify the issues that affected its future and to look at some of the options for action.

PD: And it was – I was going to say "simply" and I bet it's not easy – getting these people to come together in one room.

LW: No, it was the opposite of that! It was to use community structures that exist so you didn't have to go to all these extra meetings or get people together in one room.

It was to use the media, to use phone-in shows and television programs. It was to go into the schools. It was to really motivate all the community agencies to do what they should be doing! So for example, to the Children's Aid, we said, "Please talk about what your mandate is instead of the usual stuff you talk about."

PD: And to business, you would say?

LW: What are the issues for business in this community? Do we need new industry in this town? How are we going to provide employment? I mean, that's a perfectly legitimate and necessary thing. It was an electronic town meeting that was the connection.

PD: You were way ahead of Bill Clinton and his electronic town meetings!

LW: Well, yes. It was very widespread and the reason I say it's *apropos* is because I think we still have not learned in Canada how to involve the public in decision making. We really have no idea. We think it's by holding a meeting and people come, and five people talk, and we go home and think we've consulted.

PD: But despite their posturing, politicians and governments are afraid of people actually having their say.

LW: You better believe it! I remember, even in that process, we were pretty leery at some points. But I learned to trust the public, provided that you're perfectly transparent and the methodology and the process is clear. So we brought in resource people and so on. We had people from different systems talking to each other who would never have done that.

So when we moved to Hamilton and the church burned down the second day we were there, what we did was try to build a building which would reflect what we learned in "Town Talk." That is, how do you put together a building which will bring together people who normally don't talk to each other? Let's create a mini-community.

PD: It really is true in our culture that we tend to see "business" and "the church" as opposing each other, as not understanding each other.

LW: It wasn't always that way, but I think most of the businesspeople have now fled the church because the criticism is so strong. But in Hamilton, you see, we put the worshiping congregation at the center. We had housing for seniors, we had housing for Muslims from Egypt; there's the interfaith dimension. We had a restaurant, we had a beauty parlor, we had the outpatient clinic of the hospital. And normally, you see, you don't put a building together like that; normally, you look for the ones who can pay the most.

Although we did look for tenants who could pay well, primarily we looked for people, for entities, that normally would not interact so as to make a new style of human community.

PD: Why don't more people do that?

LW: Well, it takes a lot of energy. It takes a lot of initiative and the clue is to build trust. Who's got time to do that?

PD: Who's got time for trust?

LW: Yes, when it's easier just to ask your friends and you know...

PD: Stay in your own little circle?

LW: Stay in your own circle. It's certainly more secure.

PD: What conclusions have you reached from your world travels?

LW: As I said, I had several conversions. One was to understand that the dichotomy between the rich and the poor exists everywhere in the world, in every community, and we really need to look at that.

One of the conclusions is the theological perversion we've done with that. In *The Globe and Mail*, there was a statement which appeared three times last year: "'The poor you shall have with you always...' says so in the Bible." But that statement about the poor which Jesus made is based on an understanding of the importance of sharing and the redistribution of wealth which is present in the laws of

Deuteronomy 15, and how we have failed to abide by those laws. So the essence of what is being said is this: "The poor you shall have with you always because you do not share." So there you have the social roots of the rich and the poor.

Another one was the interfaith thing I've mentioned, realizing that Christians are a minority worldwide and that there need to be some bridges of healing there.

PD: Understanding that "respect" is an important word here.

LW: Respect and trust and also… You see, in the West, we're so given to the mode that we are the teachers, you are the learner and we will help you. There's no, or very little, thought that we have things to learn. I certainly learned that from the South Americans, Latin Americans.

PD: That they have much to teach us?

LW: They and the Asians have so much to teach us, they really have. It's cross-cultural instead of being bound up in your own little thing.

And then I have, more latterly, come into the relationships between men and women and the whole patriarchal way of looking at things and begun to understand that that has got to change as well.

PD: As we speak today, there have just been two reports released in Canada detailing the rise in racism and anti-Semitism in this country over the past year. Around the world the horror and hatred of Sarajevo carries on. We don't seem able to learn, do we?

LW: Well, we Canadians don't perceive ourselves to be racists, but, in fact, we are. One looks at the early immigration history – the Jewish ship that was sent away, the Chinese men we brought over to do all the work on the railways and then buried in some God forsaken place, what we did to the Japanese-Canadians. And we continue. I think Canada is a deeply racist country, not to mention the aboriginals and how we destroyed their culture and spirituality.

So all of that needs healing and bringing together. I find it takes a lot of energy to move into a community where you don't understand the cultural clues. But when I do that, I always learn something. Always.

PD: What's the obstacle to doing more of that?

LW: Fear, and sometimes apathy. And sometimes arrogance. After all, we're running it and we're nice people.

PD: I wondered, listening to the news reports this morning from Sarajevo, about the unfathomable depth of hatred there that survives generations.

LW: I remember the first time I was in Greece and they showed me where all the Turkish bullets had hit their walls. I asked, "Well, when was that?"
"Oh, that was 100 years ago."

PD: Is a kind of social healing possible in those situations, do you think, or is it just time that must pass?

LW: No, it isn't just time. There are attempts being made. I'm doing this project on how women are changing the liturgies and I read about one of the Asian women's gatherings where they washed each other's feet and it was an act or prayer of confession and reconciliation. For example, the Japanese who washed the Korean women's feet apologized for the Japanese government – "for my country's actions in making you Korean women prostitutes during the war." In other words, that was an act of social healing.

I don't think you'd ever find that in a Canadian setting because we don't think in those terms. But I thought that was a very strong initiative.

PD: And person-to-person.

LW: Person-to-person, but it's more than that. You take on an attitude that says, "I'm a Japanese, I'm a Canadian or whatever it is. I wasn't there personally but it's part of our history." And part of that has been the apology that churches have been making to native peoples in Canada. That's a corporate thing, that isn't just individual.

Some very nice people were running those residential schools with all the best motives in the world. But collectively, the effect was negative and so we make the apology. The native people say, "We acknowledge the apology, but we're not going to accept it until we see some change in behavior." Then that happens and we're beginning now, through the Native Healing Fund which has been established by the United Church, to make reparations. Eventually, I hope, it will be accepted.

PD: I remember being at a church/native conference in Vancouver a few years ago where the residential school experience was being discussed. A native fellow about my age started to cry when whoever it was at the podium from the church said, "We're sorry." This fellow later told me that he had to hear that apology, that there had to be a recognition of the injustice before anything else or any kind of dialogue could even be imagined.

LW: Right. But theologically, "feeling sorry" is not repentance and the native people have helped us understand that.

PD: So the route that has to then be followed is what? Increased dialogue?

LW: No! It's actions of reparation. It's restitution when possible. Then some act of reconciliation so that we begin to see each other as partners. It's a long road, a long, long road. It's a whole change in direction.

PD: You must be overwhelmed sometimes.

LW: Well, it's the way life is, the way societies are. I do think my Christian understanding of life has helped me in my social analysis of what needs to be done. And I'm not by myself. There are all sorts of people out there!

PD: So why does God allow such social injustice?

LW: Come on, I don't think God allows it. We do it apart from God!

PD: So is there a reason why we do it?

LW: Well, yes. It used to be called sin!

When people crawl on top of each other, try to put each other down and discard each other, diminish each other – it's a very human trait.

PD: But I think...

LW: Women know quite a bit about that!

PD: Behind my question was the idea that people feel disconnected from their actions and it's far easier to say, "Well, that's the way it is, that's God's fault, not mine."

LW: Oh yea, well poor God. God gets blamed for everything. I think that's a cop-out. We have done it and we need to take responsibility for it. Again, because of the individualism of our culture, we're not prepared to do that.

PD: Are you optimistic that we'll ever learn that?

LW: No! But I'm a person of hope. I think there's quite a difference between optimism and hope. If you look at the world, it's in a hell of a mess. I mean really! Wherever you look, only a fool would be optimistic.

But I'm a person of hope because I don't think that's how it is intended to be or how we are intended to live our lives.

PD: Do you think more has been accomplished in the world by anger and aggression than through love and compassion?

LW: Well, anger can be the cradle for change. It can be a strong motivating force.

PD: The energy of it?

LW: Yes, the energy of it, if it can be creatively channeled. And then it becomes love, or it can be allied to compassion. But quite often, anger is the only thing that gets us going.

PD: From your travels around the world, I wonder if there are moments or situations or experiences that stand out as guideposts for you?

LW: Oh yes! I think particularly of when I was in Chile and Argentina during the 1980s, which were the days of the dirty war when the fascist military was in charge. And in Argentina, they were simply murdering a generation of high school students and university students who were resisting a fascist government and the military.

   I got to know the mothers of May Square, as they called themselves, because every Thursday, in May Square, at their House of Parliament, they would march in twos, silently asking for news of their...

PD: Disappeared.

LW: Yea, their disappeared, which of course they never got. I mean, I know them very well. I know Juanita. I know them by name.

   The sequel to that is, of course, the grandmothers. After the dirty war, they went to work to locate their grandchildren, whom the military had kidnapped, adopted, and attempted to raise in fascist thought forms. The grandmothers located them through genetic matching and so on.

And I thought, isn't that something? The initiative they've taken! And in some instances they've been able to restore kids to their rightful parents and grandparents. That stuck with me. And yet the other thing about them is that it wasn't just an individual initiative.

I had just come from Korea where there was much of the same thing going on. The women there had given me a silver pendant, in the shape of a fish, which is the Christian symbol. On one side it said, "Jesus Christ is Lord." On the other side it said, "Set the prisoners free," because their young people were in prison. When I went to Argentina, I gave this pendant to one of the mothers of May Square. I did it on a Tuesday night in the basement of a Methodist church, because you had to meet in secret. On Thursday, I met two more of the mothers and one of them said to me, "Thank you so much for the pendant."

"I didn't give you a pendant. I'm just meeting you for the first time," I said.

"Oh," she said, "You gave it to us on Tuesday and we each get to wear it for two weeks."

I've never forgotten that because it was the solidarity of people in a caring, just relationship. That's what I'm after and I admire it so much when I see it!

PD: It must anger you that people don't see the church as a vehicle for that kind of passion, that seeking of justice.

LW: The church has not covered itself with glory in its track record in many instances. You think of the Inquisition and you think of the conquest of America – there are many things I'm very critical of when it comes to the church as an institution.

PD: But today, people don't seem to see it as the place where they can pursue that kind of justice, even if they have that spark within them.

LW: Well, because they don't see it as a place where that's happening, and, in many instances, they're right. I don't find many congregations to be hot beds of social justice, although you'll always find a core, usually a minority, that is still viable.

But, at the same time, I remember a radio interview with a fellow and we were on this subject. He was taking your line and saying, "Oh well, the church isn't really a place where you can pursue social justice anymore." I maintained that it was. And he says, "Oh yea? Listen to these congregational announcements: tomorrow we have the bazaar and on Friday we have the white elephant sale…" And I thought, oh dear, he's right.

Many people in the church discard social justice priorities in favor of bazaars and white elephant sales, which raise money for charity, not social action.

So we're a mix. We're a mix because we're people and I don't get mad at them, no. I get sad. To be involved in social justice, though, is how I've been nurtured and it seems to me to be the appropriate way for me to live my life. But I don't get mad at other people and I've got too much respect for the people in other faith communities who are doing similar things for social justice to get mad at them.

PD: Maybe I was thinking more of disappointment than anger. Are you disappointed at all?

LW: No.

PD: Because there certainly is, and I think this word is over-used, but there certainly is a "spiritual" hunger felt by many today.

LW: Yes.

PD: And I think people generally want to do well by others.

LW: Well...

PD: Am I being naive?

LW: Carry on.

PD: So while they are outraged by much of what they see in the world, they feel helpless in the face of much of it, short of writing a cheque which in the end isn't the solution.

LW: Yes, or sometimes they don't think any change is possible anyway. For example, the cynicism about the whole political process we have – what good is it going to do anyway? So they eventually retreat into their own little, private, individualistic world. On the other hand, there are numbers of people who are faithful. But they're not all in the church is my point, not by a long shot.

I mean, God works where God wants! And what you have to do is find out the signs of God's activity and join your life in that stream. Sometimes it's inside the institutional church and sometimes it's outside. So that's why I'm not angry. I'm just thankful that God is at work, that we can sometimes discern it, and that I'm able to join my life to the efforts of other people who are in those struggles.

PD: That cynicism, though, is a definite enemy to social healing isn't it?

LW: Oh yes. It means apathy. It means you can't do anything anyway. You can't trust those guys so I'm just going to build my own little tower.

PD: What do you say to people who want to exercise the kind of social concern they have but at the same time are feeling a bit cut adrift?

LW: First, you need to ally yourself with somebody else who shares similar convictions. You know, we're past the stage of heroes and heroines. It's a social movement.

What I have done is to work in social movements which I think are about transformation of our culture and transformation of our society and our world.

One is the social justice movement, one is the peace movement (which is very closely linked to the ecological movement now), one is the ecumenical movement (which is not just inter-church but is interfaith and is broader than that – it's the whole inhabited world), and one is the feminist movement (which attempts to transform the culture of patriarchy which is worldwide as well).

You soon learn that you are not the only pebble on the beach and that you can lend your energies and your spirituality. Also, you always learn in the process. So in that sense I'm a person of hope.

PD: What's the next big cultural wave that's going to hit us, do you think?

LW: I wish I knew. I wish I could answer your question, but I really can't. But I do think about it a lot. I wonder, "Why were we not aware?" I mean, how did the ecological movement arise? The signs must have been there long before we saw them. How did the feminist movement come about? The signs were there long before we became aware. And there must be something now. The signs are there but we're not discerning the signs of the times.

PD: Some suggest that the major shift taking place in the world today is one away from science, away from our dependence on the rational.

LW: Well, that's another issue that really is puzzling and there's a dichotomy there.

I'm on a federal task force for the review of the concept of disposal of nuclear waste in Canada and we get two messages from the public. One is that they have no trust in scientists. "How can we believe all that stuff you tell us?" The other is, "If we wait long enough you will find a way for us." So they have complete faith on the one hand and no faith on the other. It's a real paradox.

PD: So what do you do then?

LW: I perceive that one of the things that desperately needs to happen is to bring the scientists together with people in the humanities for a dialogue, for some conversation, because they hardly ever meet. They don't understand each other and that chasm needs to be bridged.

We're in a wildly technological society and one has to ask where is the accountability of the technology? Is it to people or is it to more technology? What is it for? Maybe that is the next cultural wave, it's upon us now.

PD: What? Seeking a balance?

LW: Well, it's the technological culture. Everybody says to me, with pity in their eyes, "Don't you have e-mail? Aren't you on e-mail?"

PD: I hate them!

LW: It's just that it's perceived that you're not really with the human race unless you're into all the slick technology, and from time to time I fall victim to that notion too.

PD: It's hard to avoid, isn't it?

LW: It's very hard to avoid and it's not all bad, to put it mildly. We owe a great deal to technology. But what is its social accountability to people and how is it being used? I think that's one of the dialogues that has really not been up front.

PD: Could you do a "Town Talk" in the 1990s?

LW: I've often thought about it. You remember when we had the constitutional talks by groups across the country linked by media? That was a kind of a half-hearted attempt at it. It wasn't broad enough, but it used some of the same principles.

Healing, obviously, has to do sometimes with surgery and I think that if I have any function, that may be it. The church would call it a prophetic point of view. It involves cutting away some things so that we're able then to see more of the truth about ourselves and about our neighbor, whether that neighbor is in Iceland or Asia or wherever, and so that healing can start. But unless and until that has happened, I think that any healing will be full of pus, it really won't work.

PD: It's cutting away, what?

LW: Cutting away our own blindness. Jesus kept saying, "Can't you hear? Can't you see? What's the matter with you people?" I think that's surgery.

So I guess healing for me is exposing oneself to situations and to people that are quite, quite different from oneself, and then listening.

PD: That takes a lot of personal energy.

LW: It takes a great deal of personal energy. It means going to that meeting and not this one. It means thinking to yourself, "I won't know a soul at this meeting; do I really want to go?"

PD: And it means being challenged, being willing to have your...

LW: Presuppositions and values challenged. Oh yes. And not fighting back, initially at least. Listening, really listening – that's hard. We're an interdependent world.

PD: I remember hearing a fellow say when the Berlin Wall came down that this was not, in Eastern Europe, a victory of ideology but a victory of consumerism.

LW: Oh yes. I often think if the States really wanted to destroy Cuba, what they should do is trade with them. Suck them in! Everybody would be buying within ten minutes. And that would be the end of Cuba.

PD: But because that consumerism seduces us into seeing the world in black and white terms, that notion leads to the idea that if you are a Christian, then you have this set of answers.

LW: Yes...

PD: And you do not have to deal with the fluidity of life.

LW: That's right. And there's really so little we know. But I think if one risks, then one finds out.

I remember, early on, Jesus' thing about it's more blessed to give than to receive. I thought that's a really peculiar thing because I just love receiving.

But I tried it, tentatively, and my own experience validated it and I thought, well I guess I can risk that again.

PD: Have you discovered anything that has really rocked your faith? As you say, you have the energy to open yourself up to new experiences.

LW: Yes.

PD: Has anything frightened you?

LW: Well, I'd say that my faith is different from when I started.

PD: In what way?

LW: In many ways.

I think it's not about belief so much as about risk. It's about putting your foot in the puddle and getting in. It's about commitment of life stance. "Frightening," I don't know.

PD: Frightening only in the sense that when the familiar ground is pulled out from beneath you...

LW: I find that exciting! I find that interesting! It means I've got some things to learn.

PD: What are you risking then?

LW: You're risking being with other people in their pain and their suffering and trusting; you're risking not having a whole lot of answers that you can trot out for every occasion; and you're risking being fully human instead of being Christian, if you can get that distinction.

PD: I think it means exactly not having all the answers.

LW: That's right. So you have to live your life on the basis of what answers you have, on the basis of what convictions you have, but, at the same time, you have to hold these convictions with an openness.

Appendix

BARBARA BISHOP is the minister of Woodbine Heights
Baptist Church in East York, Toronto. She is a member of
her own denomination's Task Force on Domestic Violence
and its Working Group on Equality in Ministry. In her community, she is a member of the East York Coalition to Stop
Violence Against Women and Children, and a member of
the Board of Directors of Alternatives, a mental health case
management agency committed to consumer/survivor par-
ticipation and extended choices for those experiencing
lengthy or significant mental health problems.

ROCHELLE GRAHAM, R.P.T., C.H.T.P., C.H.T.I., a physiotherapist for 21 years, uses Therapeutic Touch and Healing Touch in her private practice. She is certified as a Prac-
titioner and as an Instructor through the American Holistic Nurses Association. She mentors and teaches healthcare
professionals, lay people, and church members throughout
Canada and the United States.

WAYNE IRWIN, an ordained minister of the United
Church of Canada, has been in active ministry for 28 years.
He has a background in music and physics and is currently
studying the benefits for prayer practice of contemporary
studies in consciousness and thought. He is the executive
director of Lowville Prayer Centre.

JENNIFER JONAS attained a Master's degree in music therapy from Michigan State University and has developed a private practice in Toronto working with developmentally delayed children and adults as well as with the terminally ill. In 1993, Jennifer released her first digital recording entitled *Reminiscence*.

FLORA LITT is a spiritual director, trained through the Toronto School of Theology. She is an initiating member of Lowville Prayer Centre, where she serves as program manager and leads workshops in prayer, meditation, and the healing ministry with Wayne Irwin.

KATHRYN McMORROW has her own business, Innovations Seminars, and gives workshops and talks on a variety of topics in business, educational, and social service settings, in both English and French. She also teaches at McGill University. Her special area of interest is in the rapidity of change today and its effects on our well-being and productivity, in both our business and personal lives. She has done radio interviews and talk shows, as well as made television appearances in major cities across Canada.

FATHER THOMAS RYAN spent 15 years of his life at the Montreal-based Canadian Centre for Ecumenism and served as its director from 1984–1995. He is currently the director of Unitas. He has authored six books in the areas of spirituality and ecumenism including, *Prayer of Heart and Body: Meditation and Yoga as Christian Spiritual Practice; Wellness,*

Spirituality and Sports; Fasting Rediscovered: A Guide to Health and Wholeness for Your Body-Spirit.

DONNA SINCLAIR is a writer/journalist who lives in North Bay, Ontario. She is a senior writer with *The United Church Observer* and her particular areas of interest include faith and spirituality, native people, children, and justice issues. The author of seven books, she is currently working on *A Woman's Book of Days* for Northstone Publishing, Inc. She taught creative writing at Canadore College for 12 years, and has won awards both for fiction and for articles in categories ranging from news coverage to devotional/inspirational to editorial courage. Alone or with her husband, Jim Sinclair, she's led workshops on a wide variety of topics, including Christian parenting, angels, and dreams.

JIM SINCLAIR has been a minister at St. Andrew's United Church in North Bay, Ontario, since 1979. He has accompanied people on their spiritual journeys, both as a pastor and as a human rights activist in Canada, South Africa, and Central America. A trained counselor, Jim has been a supervisor in Clinical Pastoral Education (CPE), and since the mid-1970s has worked with people in both CPE programs and in the internship program of the United Church. He has served as chair both of the executive of the United Church's national Judicial Committee, and of the national Candidature Committee. For the past 30 years, he and his wife, Donna Sinclair, have co-led workshops on many subjects, including – for the past 17 years – dreams.

KELLY WALKER is a popular Canadian public speaker. He has inspired audiences throughout North America on the Can*Speak circuit. He has had a private practice mainly for professionals working through burnout issues. He is on the international training team for Rainbows, a program for children facing grief or divorce in their family. He is a founding member of Sacred Acts, a school for the performing arts. He is also a celebrated singer-songwriter and recording artist. He lives in the heart of downtown Toronto.

LOIS WILSON has been moderator of the United Church of Canada, as well as president of the Canadian Council of Churches. Her position as president of the World Council of Churches (1983–1991) provided the impetus and opportunity for extensive global travel. She is currently chancellor of Lakehead University. Lois has written four books including *Like a Mighty River* and *Turning the World Upside Down,* and is currently working on a fifth book for Northstone Publishing, Inc.